A better Life with Parkison's
Through Ayurveda & Yoga

Raja Ray

PREVENTION MANAGEMENT SELF-HELP

Note:

The information contained in this book is presented to the best of our knowledge and has been checked with the utmost care.

Since this information cannot replace the advice of a competent specialist but can merely supplement it, it is recommended that any user consult a doctor. The author and publisher accept no liability for damages or consequences resulting from the use or misuse of the information presented here.

Table of Contents

Dedication v
Thanksgiving vi
Foreword vii
How to use This Book xi
Introduction xiii

PART 1 - PREVENTION 1

Chapter 1: Patient Stories 3
Chapter 2: Yoga and Parkinson's 17
Chapter 3: Yoga Therapy and Ayurveda 25
Chapter 4: Yoga & Ayurveda
Lifestyle for Parkinson's Patients 41

PART 2 - MANAGEMENT 51

Chapter 5: Self-Confidence 53
Chapter 6: Spirituality 55
Chapter 7: Parkinson's Yoga 59
    Yoga for the mobile patient (YOGA I) 62
    Yoga at the chair for patients with
    movement hints (YOGA II) 99

PART 3 - SELF-HELP 121

Chapter 8: Practical Solutions for Parkinson's Patients 123
    Living with tremors 123
    Dealing with muscle stiffness 123
    Yoga dancing and Parkinson's 123

Stand up, sit down, turn to the side.. 124
Help with walking... 124
Improving swallowing capacity...125
Falling 125
Depression..125
Pain and mental immobility 126
Problem management 126
    a. Small steps... 126
    b. Freezing..127
    c. Tremors...127
    d. Drooling and swallowing problems 127
    e. Standing up from a chair 127
    f. Depression...127

Chapter 9: Clinical Procedure.. 129
Chapter 10: Letters From Patients..133

Conclusion...137

This book is dedicated to
Prof. Dr. Horst Przuntek
from whom I learned about Parkinson's.

THANKS to

All of my patients, who were my family, friends and German teachers,

And special thanks to:

The late Dr. Mass (Berlin)
The late Mr. Niermann (Bern)
Mr. Vossbrink (Bochum)
Mrs. Kables (Hamburg)
Mr. Feustel (Cologne)
Mr. Ehm (Essen)
Mrs. Lore Tomalla (Cologne)
Christiane Elle (Product Designer)

Forward

In a Protestant hospital in Germany is a medical department for Neurology and Complimentary Medicine supported by the state. The department is headed by Professor Horst Przuntek. In this 20-bed Neurological Ward for Modern Medicine, Ayurveda and yoga therapy work together.

I first worked as a yoga teacher and as an Ayurvedic Therapist. In the year 2008, I was working with a luxury 5-star hotel in Goa. The hotel was equipped with helipads, a golf course, and a beach. I worked there as a yoga teacher.

In November, a hotel guest offered me a job after learning yoga with me for two weeks. This guest, Professor Przuntek, wanted me to make a new yoga therapy for those with Parkinson's Disease. As he was going to open a new station for Neurology and Complimentary Medicine in Germany, he wanted to integrate Ayurveda and yoga with modern medicine. Prof. Przuntek was one of the best neurologists for Parkinson's in Germany. He had written more than 500 scientific papers in international science journals.

Though I have worked with yoga and Ayurvedic therapy for five years in different clinics in India, Parkinson's and Neurology were totally new to me. But the task was interesting and challenging, so on May 4th of 2009, with only two German words which I learned five minutes before, I started my yoga class. I was 28 years old, and all my Patients were over 60.

For about three years, I taught yoga to twenty patients every day. I also led six daily Ayurvedic physical therapy sessions. I worked eight and a half hours per day, totaling 42 hours per week. During my time in the Neurology ward, I've taught and worked with more than 500 patients, most of whom came from Europe. Some were from Asia and the Arabic countries of the Middle East. My patients ranged in age from 23 to 87. Some were gay or lesbian, and some had fought in World War II. Their occupations varied widely as well; I treated everyone from businessmen to tango dancers, truck drivers to students, Catholic priests to nurses, TV journalist to asylum seekers, and dentist to psychologists.

Some used wheelchairs, and others were psychologically demented. I worked with patients who had all kinds of motor disorders; everything from restless legs to expressionless faces to small handwriting. Our neurological ward was a very normal department supported by the Krankenkasse, German's social health insurance. Patients liked to come again and again. Every day, they had morning yoga, a medical visit, Ayurvedic therapies, physical therapy, psychological counseling, speech therapy, occupational therapy, and Ayurvedic food to eat.

The quality of life gradually improved for most of our patients. During their stay, they worked on their motor functions, balance, coordination, cognitive abilities, smelling capacity, and made gains in their overall health. Some patients came with a walking stick but left without the need for one, able to live a new life.

This book's objective is to help Parkinson's patients find a different viewpoint towards Parkinson's Disease. I also want to share my practical knowledge that I gained through my everyday experiences. Parkinson's patients are wonderful people, creative and strong. Some of them have invited me to their homes, where I stayed with them, and learned from them; I'd like to share these experiences in this book.

This book is not a medicinal book or a substitute to Parkinson's therapy. It is simply meant to convey the experiences of patients who used Ayurveda and yoga to improve their quality of life.

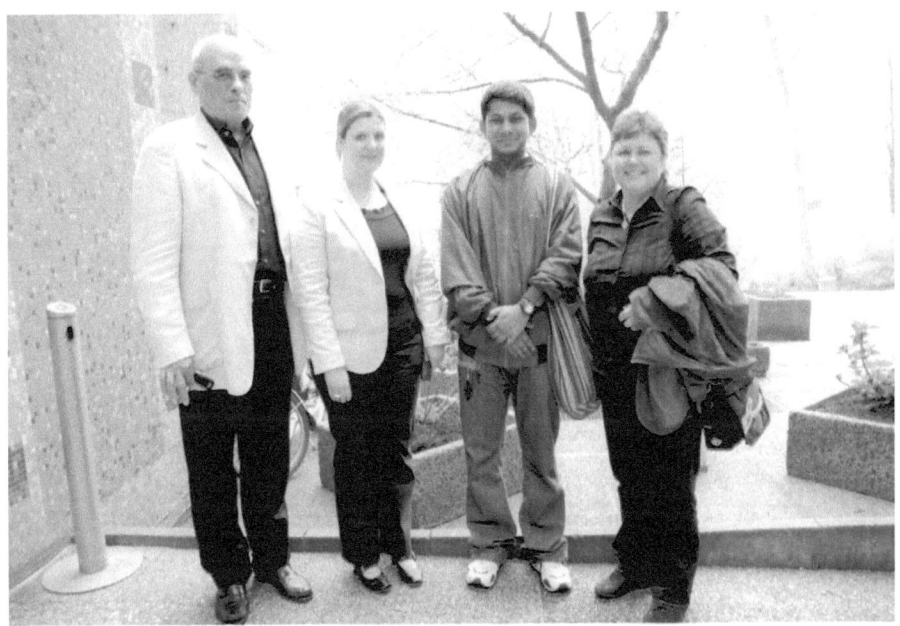

My first day with Professor Przuntek and his German colleagues.

How to Use this Book

Apart from my work with yoga, I used to give Ayurvedic massages and therapies to all my patients. Through this book, I cannot even give you a feet, back, or head massage, but you can read and hopefully enjoy the stories thoughts shared here.

Alas, you have to do and read all alone. If one wants to directly start to Exercise in morning, evening or any time that is comfortable; please start with Chapter 7 with Yoga Program 2, Sitting in a Chair with comfortable loose dressing, Start with simple movements. Then one can Proceed to Yoga 1 program. Please give a gap of 2 hours after eating heavy meal like lunch or dinner. Do what you can, do not force, main thing is you enjoy the movements.

The Book is divided into 3 parts, Prevention, Management and Self-help. Starting with chapter 1 with Stories of patients to contemplate with, chapter 2 is How Yoga and Parkinson is connected, Chapter 3 deals with little scientific background of Yoga Therapy Ayurveda and its benefits, Chapter 4 is about the outline of a Yoga & Ayurveda Lifestyle diet concept that leads towards healing Chapter 5 is about Motivation and confidence, Chapter 6 is about Spiritual tools to get inner peace, Chapter 8 is about some guidelines solving daily problems with movement, Chapter 9 is about the Clinical concept of our Medical Team and last chapter 10 is about what patients got benefit and relief, so I share their personal Letters with you..

I wrote this book with patients in mind; I did not want to make this book thick or complicated, a story only for scientific community. I wanted to share stories that are simple and funny, experiences that I hope will be relatable and enjoyable to Parkinson's patients.

I have intentionally removed the technical language and medical complexities from this book in order to make it more engaging and digestible for all Parkinson's patients.

I hope that one day, I can meet you all personally and laugh together. Perhaps then, you can stick your tongue out at me to improve the fine motor skills, articulation, and facial expression as we share laughter together through face yoga.

Enjoy the book and the stories of my experiences.

Introduction

In the mind there is binding (prison) & in the mind there is freedom. The mind only knows truly that you are weak or strong.
-Vam Dev(Tarapeet)

When you have severe pain in your knee that restricts your normal movement due to arthritis and someone tells you that he will replace your knee with a metal one, you'd likely be quite afraid. But if a doctor says that he will replace your knee, then you will believe him and go in for a operation without truly knowing whether it will be successful or not.

A normal person does not know modern medicine, but he still believes in it. It is this trust and acceptance that comes from the mind; the mind is therefore the greatest medicine. Yoga, an Indian philosophy, has recognized this for thousands of years. Yoga therefore refers to the union of body, mind, and soul. Most diseases come from the mind. Unbalanced stress translates into sicknesses like heart attacks, ulcers, or diabetes and weaken our immune systems. People have complicated their lives with anger, greed, lust, jealousy, and egos; yoga gives us guidance on making our lives simple.

Disease originates from indigestion—not only indigestion of food but also indigestion of thoughts, emotions, and suppressed behavior. Then the toxins remain, resulting in constipation. Ayurvedic medicine teaches that constipation is the mother of all diseases; it results in a fat belly which in turn leads to improper breathing. Improper breathing leads to fatigue, dull skin, eyes, and a dull life.

Then these toxins translate into arthritis, and they pollute the blood, mind, and even the soul. We drag our bodies around like living corpses until we die with a deformed, diseased body. We age with disgrace. My interest is in the quality of dying.

Dogs typically live for their full life span, 12 years, and sometimes they live even longer. A human's potential life span is one hundred and fifty years. But most of us die at the age of 70 or 80. Why? It's not just drugs and alcohol; our complicated relationship with food and the way we live our lives are also responsible.

If you go to visit a new city, you typically buy a tourist guide or map first, and then you choose which church or museum you will visit, what roads you will take, and which places to avoid. Yoga, like a map, is a guide for life management. It provides you tools with which you can create your own software, allowing you to develop a program for running your own health and healing your body.

Be your own light.
-Indian Proverb

Self-help is the best help. God helps those who help themselves. Just as a small seed grows into a tree, humans can provide the seed with a good environment, water, and fertilizers, but it's the tree's own struggle to survive and grow. It is up to him how he will use the sunlight and air to spread branches and leaves.

As doctors, yoga teachers, and therapists, we can give medicine, recommend life styles, and provide therapy, but it is up to the patient to determine how to grow into health and healing.

Yoga and Ayurveda will help you find your inner program for health and healing.

grow into health and healing

PART 1 –
PREVENTION

Prevention is the best cure for any illness. Go to sleep early and eat healthy foods. Save your energy by talking less and making your mind empty through meditation. Smile, laugh, whistle, and do yoga every day. Movement is the key to life, and it is what will keep you alive.

Chapter 1: Patient Stories

The patients in the hospital served as my family, friends, and guides. They had different ages, different social backgrounds, and were typically of a different nationality than my own. It was quite an interesting way for me to get to know a new culture and country. These patients were my German teachers, and I was their yoga teacher and Ayurveda therapist.

I often sang with them and also was invited often to cook Ayurvedic food in their houses. My patients even organized yoga workshops for me. I was invited to both weddings and funerals.

Many other personal interactions helped me get to know the lives and feelings of my patients. I was able to gain insight into their living and healing. The existence of these wonderful people was a gift to me, and I want to share some stories from our time together. For privacy purposes, I am changing their names and the finer details of their identities.

Lars

Lars was a young German man of 50 with long hair. He looked like a rock star, and he always wore long shoes made from snake's skin. Whenever he came to the hospital, Lars brought roses for the whole department. If we saw red roses, we knew Lars was there.

He wanted to become a Formula One driver, but due to his Parkinson's disease, he couldn't pursue that dream. Instead, he started a small firm that restored old sports cars. His motto was "Life is just racing; what happens before and after is just waiting."

Lars slowed down over the years. Though he was diagnosed young, he did not take any modern medicine for 15 years. He had tried many alternative methods, and after hearing about modern medicine and complimentary medicine working together, he decided to give this treatment option a chance.

Lars was so slow in his moments that he used to joke that he was a robot without the batteries.

I first met Lars in my second yoga class of the day, which was a class for chair yoga. His movements were so slow that he couldn't rotate his fingers properly. After a week of treatment from our team, however, he was able to attend my larger yoga session and master some advanced movements.

After fifteen years of slow movement, it took Lars only twenty-one days to improve dramatically. By his last day, he was so much better that he gifted me a ride in a sports car that his firm had restored. When his son came to meet his father, Lars opened the passenger door for me and took over the driver's seat. He drove to the nearest highway, and the speedometer showed us going over 300 Km.

I was a little nervous, but he had all the fun that he could have.

When he left the hospital, Lars was a new man, and he looked forward to- a life filled with new confidence and hope. In the fifteen years Lars had been affected by the disease, his technicians had left his company, and they took many of his old customers with them. They had said that Lars had no chance of succeeding in his business. Now that Lars had his health and speed back, he worked hard to start new projects and expand his business again.

He used to visit our Clinic- when he was tired, Our Clinic became an Rehabilitation Centre for Him.

Our Professor once said to Lars" Lars you are Still Young, Save your health that you gained; If you speed so much you will burn out fast."

Claudia

Just imagine- dancing throughout the night with a Parkinson's patient in a disco in a big German city.

Claudia arranged a yoga workshop for me in a river-front city. I had wanted to visit that city for a while and enjoy a quiet escape from my hectic work schedule in the hospital, so I accepted her invitation.

After finishing the yoga workshop, Claudia invited me to a revolving glass-top restaurant located in a high tower in the middle of the city. From there, we had a panoramic view of the dark city with lights all over and the river flowing like a wine stream.

After having a couple of cocktails Claudia opened her heart to me. I learned that she had two sons and, at fifty-two, had been divorced for more than a decade. I asked her why she got separated from her husband, and she told me that her husband had wanted to control her life. He didn't want to enjoy himself the way she did; he said Claudia wasn't grown up and just behaved like a teenager, not taking enough responsibility for family life.

Her oldest son, Noah, was twenty-five and was working towards a Master's degree. She was proud of him, Claudia told me. Noah was self-sufficient, able to manage his life without his father's presence.

But her younger son, Jonathan, was a daddy's boy. He was still in school, and Claudia felt that he needed his father's touch in everything. He used to meet with his father once a month, but Claudia's ex-husband was a depressed and lonely person. As a result, Jonathan started to withdraw from the outside world. He stopped going to school and playing outside. He played video games throughout the day on the internet, only interacting with his virtual friends. Eventually, Claudia had to put her son in a rehab clinic for teenagers.

Now, she needed money to pay for Jonathan's rehab. She had been working half-days as a counselor in a women's support group. Her eighty-one year-old mother used to give her some money for her grandchildren, but nowadays her mother is no longer clear in the head. Claudia said that when she visited her mother's home, her mother would just talk about wanting to die. I learned that she has been admitted to a hospital. For a while, Claudia and her sister were nursing her mother during the daytime, alternating days.

Then, her sister had a sudden stroke. Her left side was left paralyzed, and Claudia was all alone in taking care of her family. Her older son contributed some money, and Claudia had to work full-time for the income. She had to sell her car as well. Her car, Claudia told me, had been her one protected place because her home life was so difficult. Now, her only escape was dancing on weekends and sometimes spending the night with men.

As a therapist, I wanted to tell her not to dance through the night on weekends, to sleep more and strengthen her nervous system. But as a visitor, I couldn't tell her to stop one of her only remaining forms of relaxation and fun.

Dr. Schmidt

Dr. Schmidt, another man who regularly came to our clinic, took a special liking to me. To him, I was an exotic young man. He was a retired nuclear scientist who lived with a dentist named Michael. Dr. Schmidt had a daughter from his earlier marriage, and his daughter used to say that she had two fathers.

It all started with a disturbance in the left eyeball and left side of Dr. Schmidt's face. Gradually, his body began to lean to the left side, and his walk was unstable.

I spent my first Christmas and New Year's in Germany at Dr. Schmidt's home in Berlin. He frequently held parties in his huge apartment, as he had an affinity for socializing. On December 31st at midnight, we all went to the rooftop garden of his apartment. We lifted our wine glasses to the Berlin sky and cheered to the stars above.

I met wonderful people at the doctor's parties. I met therapists from Thailand, cooks from Sri Lanka, and everyone in between. Their commonalities were found in music and food. At these parties, Michael played his grand piano, and Dr. Schmidt played the violin.

Dr. Schmidt also planned my Europe trip when my family came over from India. I visited him every Christmas, and for years, all was well. However, after several years, a pain from his lower back spread towards his legs. He could no longer sleep well at night or walk properly. He opted for spinal surgery, but it worsened the situation.

He wanted to live his life fully until the end. I said to him, "You are focusing on external stimulation, your likes and dislikes, but you're not respecting and protecting the life within your body." For example, his bedroom was up a flight of stairs, so I suggested that he sleep in the guest room on the first floor instead. Similarly, he used to walk down to the city center, taking small and unstable steps, to eat in vegan restaurants. He often lost his balance and fell in the streets, cutting his forehead and covering his elbows with bruises. I suggested that he order food in instead.

Once, I was with Dr. Schmidt when he fell. I called an ambulance, and we rushed to an emergency ward. He was bleeding seriously, but at the time, his only concern was whether the ambulance expenses would be covered by his medical insurance.

After that, I suggested that he only walk inside his home and that he use a wheelchair when he left the house. He told me that he could still walk and wasn't ill — he refused to use a wheelchair at all.

Though his health was deteriorating, Dr. Schmidt still liked to invite people to his apartment during Christmas and New Year's. Throughout the year, Dr. Schmidt lived strictly according to the health standard prescribed by the clinic, but towards the end of December, he filled his time with people, food, wine, and fun. Michael wasn't crazy about having so many people over; he figured that so much excitement was worse for Dr. Schmidt's health.

Doctors suspected that Dr. Schmidt had colon cancer, but he wasn't formally diagnosed. His intestine became sensitive, and he could no longer digest food. Slowly, his body collapsed in on itself in a hospital.

I received an invitation for the funeral in the mail, It was very painful for me .... I did not want to go. But I had not seen him for many months. So I decided to go and pay my last respects.

Oliver

Oliver was a sports journalist. He used to anchor a television program, about the latest high-end sports cars. He had been hosting the program for decades, so he was something of a television star. At first, Oliver hid his disease, afraid he would lose his television job, but he finally had to step down as the symptoms worsened.

He had a special aura about him, and he aroused the attention of many of our patients. Even the young female nurses had a soft spot for Oliver. He looked quite smart, but upon close observation, one could see that Oliver's chin was close to his upper chest. His neck protruded oddly, and one of his shoulders was unusually stiff. Oliver had been married and had two daughters, but he divorced after his wife found a new love in Australia and settled there. When I met him, Oliver had a steady girlfriend who cared for him and helped him manage his Parkinson's. However, I learned that he also had many affairs.

Once, a girl with whom Oliver had a one night stand called his girlfriend and told her that the two of them had slept together. Oliver's girlfriend confronted him, asking whether it had really happened.

Oliver convinced his girlfriend that the Parkinson's medicine increased his sex drive and that he couldn't control himself, mitigating the damage to his relationship.

He was a nice guy to talk to. Often during breaks in our therapy sessions, we would talk about sports and the car industry. When

I visited him in his room, I often founded him chatting on a dating website, looking for casual sex.

He used to write articles for journals throughout the night or chat online with girls he didn't know. He regularly arrived late to his therapy session. More than once, I went to his room in the morning and found him sleeping on his laptop at the table in the corner. A few times, I saw different girls leaving his room, his hospital bed sheets disheveled. I heard from Professor secretary that Oliver had invited a beautiful young Turkish Nurse to spend her holiday in Mallorca with him at his private house.

I did not understand why he was living like this. Was he frustrated about his life? As he was not in the Television Show. Why he is using his Medicines as an excuse to have more sex? Even making sex in the hospital bed. Not sleeping in nights. Just thinking by just staying for 21 days in this Clinic can Heal him.

Dieter and Alex

Dieter was a 51 year multiple sclerosis (MS) patient. He was suffering from MS for 15 years and had lost his job as a firefighter before he came to the clinic. His wife had left him for another man, and his small child didn't understand why her father could no longer play with her.

Dieter used to walk with a stick. He was always angry — he came across as rude and arrogant to me. When he first came to our clinic, he refused to follow the prescribed vegetarian diet. But he attended my Yoga II class, "Chair Yoga," in one corner of the hospital floor. He used to hold his stick in one hand and hold onto the wall or chair as he did his yoga movements.

Eventually, he wanted to attend Yoga I, which was for patients who could sit on the floor and try normal yoga movements without the help of a chair. After two years at our clinic, he became a different man. He walked without a stick, and over time he became friendlier, eventually smiling in greeting.

Another patient suffering from MS was Alex, a twenty-two year old man. He had been studying computer programming when he was diagnosed, and at the time, he had been dating a girl named Anna for more than seven years. Six months after he was diagnosed, he came to our clinic.

Alex often wore a cap turned backwards, and I could just see a tattoo protruding from his wrist to the upper part of his hand. He always had Bob Marley and reggae music playing on his iPhone. He often went down to the hotel lobby to smoke or drink a Coca Cola. Although he was much like other young men in these regards, his upper body curved, and he stooped as he walked, his steps slow and labored.

He easily accepted the clinic's vegetarian diet, but he didn't want to try Ayurvedic therapies. It took persuasion from his girlfriend before he began to try manual therapies.

The doctors also wanted to inject cortisone into his spinal fluid, but Alex refused. It was easy to understand why he was hesitant — no one enjoys spinal injections in the lower back. But he was turning down what the doctors saw as one of his best options.

Other than this, Alex still attended my Chair Yoga class on occasions. He and I talked about yoga philosophy and shared our viewpoints on life; over time, we became good friends.

At one point, Alex came to the hospital and told me that his girlfriend was pregnant. I was amazed that such a young girl would choose to have a baby with a diseased man. I had a lot of respect for Anna.

When I visited Alex, I often saw Anna's swollen belly as she helped clear his dishes from the dining table. Alex was lucky that, even in the advanced stages of pregnancy, his girlfriend was still willing to tend to him with so much care.

Six months after I learned that Anna was pregnant, Alex came to the hospital and announced that he was the father of a beautiful baby girl. He stood in the common eating space to make an announcement, and the patients around him cheered. My heart was filled with joy.

Alex and Anna got married, and a year later, they had a baby boy.

But as time passed, Alex's body became stiffer. The doctors had to give him oral medicine. He still refused spinal injections, and I could no longer persuade him to attend my yoga sessions.

Alex invited me to his house for his daughter's birthday. While there, I learned that Anna worked as a midwife while Alex stayed at home writing letters to Social Security, looking to get money from the State. According to the government, Alex was still capable of working from home because he had studied computer sciences, but instead, he listened to music and used marijuana weekly to calm himself down. It seemed to me that he had no interest in working, at home or otherwise.

Later, I asked my professor about his views on marijuana. He say that it may do some initial good, but in long run, its effects on the liver and nervous system outweigh the benefits. Additionally, it can become increasingly addictive over time, and it can cause memory and cognition problems. The professor also mentioned the risk of children taking it by accident.

I found it odd that Dieter and Alex, both of whom had multiple sclerosis, took such different paths over the years. Dieter was older and had a less pleasant disposition when he started treatment, but his health improved. Alex was a young guy with two little children who was getting all the support he could from his wife, but his condition deteriorated.

Peter

Two of our patients were a nice elderly German couple. The woman was fit enough to push her husband's wheelchair, and they would sometimes come to my morning yoga class.

The man, Peter, was very thin; his rib bones protruded through the skin, and his body was so curved that he looked as though he was reverting to a fetus, his head spiraling inwards towards his stomach. He sat on his wheelchair, unable to move his joints. Peter couldn't talk, and his face had a blank look, but he clearly had full consciousness and understood my voice.

I used to tell him to try to move his various body parts, and that if he couldn't, to imagine moving the body part anyways.

One of the exercises I had patients do in my yoga class was to laugh in three different ways. When it was Peter's turn, he couldn't move his face muscles, although he was trying hard. A tear drop ran down his face.

I simply moved on and asked the next patient to take her turn.

The next morning, Peter didn't come to yoga, so I went to his room to check on him. The senior neurological doctors were there for their daily morning visit when I arrived. His wife told them that Peter was making a strange sound through his throat and could only manage labored breathing through his mouth. The doctors said that they would send for some tests of Peter's wind pipe.

I knew that a medical test would be uncomfortable for Peter; it would entail inserting a device in his throat. I felt that his diaphragm was tight, and I figured that his lungs and heart weren't getting enough space in his ribcage. So I asked the doctors to hold off on Peter's test for a couple days.

I modified a yoga posture that opens the diaphragm so that Peter could do it in his hospital bed. I helped him hold the posture, using the pillows as props. After a few minutes, his breathing was normal. He closed his mouth and was able to breathe through his nose; the stage sound was gone. Not long after that, he went to sleep.

Though I cannot communicate with him as he cannot speak and he cannot move his body to show some body language, So that I can understand. But still the Yoga posture communicated with him.

Peter continued using this pose to relax, and within a few days, his face was bright again. He even started to smile, and in my yoga class, he was able to show three different kinds of laughter.

Joachim Siegburg

Joachim couldn't keep his head still, and it used to bounce around as though just his head was dancing, his long white beard flopping from side to side. By taking medicine, he could sometimes keep his head still, but when the medicine wore off, his head started to move again.

The quality of his movements improved with Ayurveda and yoga therapies. He could turn and roll in his bed again. A pain that he'd had in his right arm for thirty years vanished. Joachim said that these treatments helped with his overall health, not just his Parkinson's. After Joachim learned more about Ayurvedic medicine, he asked for treatment for his erectile dysfunction, so it helped his love life too.

Joachim was also a great admirer of furniture design. He had an amazing collection of model chairs from all over the world. I was also interested in art and design, so we bonded over several visits to museums in Switzerland and Germany.

When I moved to a new apartment, he did the interior design and even helped me carry the furniture and lights from Ikea. I couldn't fix my bed frame, and I asked him for help. Even though he had to go to the dentist for an operation the next day, he came to help.

I also cooked Ayurvedic food for him regularly, and he told me that he found it both tasty and healthy. Whenever he got bored of the hospital food, he used to bring a fellow patient with him to my apartment, and we would all eat together.

He invited me to spend the Easter holidays with him in Switzerland. After playing Pétanque with him, we went for a walk by the side of the river Aare with his dog, Arko.

Joachim told me that he used to have a furniture shop that he had inherited from his father along with lots of debts. His father left him with so many financial problems that he couldn't pay them back until he turned fifty-five.

His stress increased as he worked to pay off the debt, and finally he had to sell the furniture shop to repay his father's debts. He couldn't save much, and he didn't pay enough towards his pension fund. In these hard times, he developed Parkinson's.

He had to retire early and got some money from Social Security.

At first, he thought Parkinson's was his enemy, the worst enemy he would ever have to deal with. Parkinson's had invaded his life; it took up more space than even his wife, as it came, unwanted, into his body. And eventually, this affair with Parkinson's resulted in his divorce.

He was left alone, defeated, and depressed. Eventually, Joachim's best friend asked him to spend a few weeks with him in Madeira, a beautiful island in Portugal. There, he found the new love of his life, Mirium.

Mirium, who was also divorced, was a librarian in a small Swiss city.

She found his dancing head very funny. She even trusted in his driving abilities though his head moved; he could still drive perfectly. They drove over the hills watching birds and butterflies, and at the beach, they jumped into the ocean waves.

Her family did not approve of their relationship. Her friends thought there was no future to their relationship. Joachim was ill and unproductive. It made sense to be sympathetic, they thought, but not to have a relationship with him.

Yet every weekend, Mirium travelled from Switzerland to Germany to meet Joachim, since he didn't have money to travel.

Joachim had nothing left in Germany. His shop and his family were no longer there. So eventually, he moved to Switzerland and lived with Mirium in her home. She bought a dog to walk alongside the River Aare with him.

He began to collect stones from the riverbed and painted with them. He gifted me some of these paintings, and he eventually became quite famous from his art exhibitions.

Joachim had lost everything in his life: his business, family, health and even his country. But Parkinson's gave his life back. It's funny, but with his disease, he found a new love, a new source of creativity, and a new profession.

There are many more stories that I can share with. Hope in future if I ever do Yoga Workshops with Parkinson patients - I would like to tell those stories.

a new love, a new source of creativity, and a new profession.

Chapter 2: Yoga and Parkinson's

One of my Parkinson's patients said "I am living with a thief in my body. It controls all of my functions: my visual perceptions, cognition, blood pressure, body temperature, and my sex life. It takes away my dignity — I'm losing all my motor skills and the power to control my life."

Can we control our bodies? We tend to think so, but do we have control over our heartbeats or pulses? Can we decide when we're born and when we die?

It is in facing the question of control over our bodies that yoga and Parkinson's intersect.

Yoga is not just the stretching and relaxation exercises that one finds in gyms. Yoga is a tool to improve one's lifestyle. It brings balance and harmony to the physical, mental, emotional, and spiritual dimensions of each practitioner's personality, so we can interact with our society in a better way.

Power to control my life.

What is Parkinson's?

Parkinson's disease is a progressive neurological disorder. Its symptoms vary, and not all people are severely disabled. The disorder affects a small portion of brain and is characterized by tremor, stiffness, and slowness of movements. It progresses gradually, and symptoms include a stooped posture, an expression less face, speech problems, drooling, and problems with dexterity.

In contrast to many other neurological disorders, the nature of the brain degeneration that produces Parkinson's disease has been well understood for decades. The symptoms are caused by loss of nerve cells which, for reasons that are not fully understood, are especially vulnerable to damage of various shorts, including drugs, disease, and head trauma. This malfunction is triggered by shortage of dopamine, one of the chemicals that transmit messages between nerves. Research for treatment has focused on either replacing or stimulating diminished supplies of dopamine with potent drugs, most notably L-dopa.

History

Symptoms of Parkinson's disease have been known and treated since medieval times, most notably by Averroes. However, the disease was not formally recognized and its symptoms were not documented until in 1817 in "An Essay on the Shaking Palsy" by the British physician James Parkinson's. Parkinson's disease was then known as *paralysis agitans*; the term "Parkinson's disease" was later coined by Jean -Martin Charcot.

The underlying biochemical changes in the brain were identified in 1950, largely due to the work of Swedish scientist Arvid Carlsson, who later went on to win a Nobel Prize. L-dopa entered clinical practice in 1967, and the first large study reporting improvements in patients with Parkinson's disease patients treated with L-dopa was published in 1968.

Symptoms

Parkinson's disease has both motor symptoms and non-motor symptoms.

Motor symptoms, the cardinal symptoms, are:
- Tremors: Normally 4-6 Hz tremors, maximal when the limb is at rest, and decreased with voluntary movement. It is typically unilateral at onset. This is the most apparent and well-known symptom, though an estimated 30% of patients have few perceptible tremors.
- Rigidity: Stiffness, increased muscle tone. In combination with a resting tremor, this produces rigidity when the limb is passively moved.
- Ankinesia/Bradykinesia: Absence of movement and slowness, respectively. Rapid, repetitive movements produce a dysrhythmic loss of amplitude.
- Postural instability: Failure of postural reflexes, which leads to impaired balance and falls.

Other motor symptoms include:
- Gait and posture disturbances such as shuffling, stooping, festination, gait "freezing,"
- Speech disturbances such as hypophonia (soft speech), monotonic speech, and intelligible speech
- Drooling: most likely caused by weak, infrequent swallowing and stooped posture
- Dysphagia: impaired ability to swallow. Can lead to aspiration pneumonia.
- fatigue
- Hypomimia: A mask-like face characterized by stillness and infrequent blinking;
- Difficulty rolling in bed or rising from a seated position
- Micrographia: small,cramped handwriting
- Impaired gross motor coordination
- Akathisia: the inablity to sit still
- Oily skin and seborrheic dermatitis
- Urinary incontinence,typically in later disease progression

- Nocturia(getting up in the night to pass urine)-up to 60% of cases
- Constipation and gastric dysmotility that is severe enough to endanger comfort and health

Parkinson's disease also causes cognitive and mood disturbances. Seventy percent of individuals with Parkinson's disease diagnosed with pre-existing anxiety subsequently develop depression, apathy or abulia.

Cognitive disturbances include:
- Slowed reaction time; both voluntary and involuntary motor responses are significantly slowed.
- Executive dysfunction, characterized by difficulties in allocation of attention, impulse control, prioritizing, or evaluating
- Dementia: a later development in approximately 20-40% of all patients, typically starting with the slowing of thought and progressing to difficulties with abstract thought, memory and behavioral regulation. Hallucinations, delusions and paranoia may develop.
- Short term memory loss; procedural memory is more impaired than declarative memory. Prompting elicits improved recall.
- Non-motor causes of speech/language disturbance in both expressive and receptive language. These disturbances include decreased verbal fluency and cognitive disturbance especially related to comprehension of emotional content of speech and of facial expression.
- Difficulty deceiving others, a problem that links to prefrontal hypometabolism.
- Excessive daytime somnolence
- Initial, intermediate, or terminal insomnia
- Disturbances in REM sleep: disturbingly vivid dreams, and REM Sleep Disorder, characterized by acting-out of dream

content. It can occur years prior to diagnosis.
- Impaired visual contrast sensitivity, spatial reasoning, colour discrimination, convergence insufficiency (characterized by double vision) and oculomotor control
- Dizziness and fainting, usually attributable orthostatic hypotension, a failure of the autonomic nervous system to adjust blood pressure in response to changes in body position
- Impaired proprioception (the awareness of bodily position in three-dimensional space)
- Reduction or loss of sense of smell (hyposmia or anosmia); can occur years prior to diagnosis
- Pain: attributable to tension, dystonia, rigidity, joint stiffness, and injuries associated with attempts at accommodation
- Altered sexual function, characterized by profound impairment of sexual arousal, behavior, orgasm, and drive; found in mid and late Parkinson's diseases.

Ayurveda

Ayurveda is a Traditional Indian Medicine (TIM) originating from India. "Ayur-" means life and "-veda" means knowledge. Therefore, Ayurveda means Knowledge of Life.

Ayurveda says constipation is the mother of all diseases, so it operates under the belief that diseases start from intestines. Modern research in Germany also generally concurs; it indicates that Parkinson's starts in the intestine as early as twelve years before it manifests in other ways.

Mucuna pruriens is a plant of the legume family that has been used by Ayurvedic Practitioners to treat Parkinson's for more than 4,500 years; Western medicine is now accepting mucuna as an alternative treatment to, or complementary therapy with, L-dopa. Research cited by the National Parkinson's Foundation found that

"Dose to dose, mucuna was two to three times more effective than equivalent amounts of synthetic drugs."

Ayurvedic medicine and the fourteen to twenty-one day Ayurvedic detoxification program can particularly help Parkinson's patients. These programs, which last only a few weeks, can help patients feel better and improve their qualities of life.

Parkinson's and Yoga

Parkinson's is a movement disorder disease, and although it primarily shows itself through motor symptoms, it can also affect behavior, thinking, and sensations. Its main symptoms are stiffness, rigidity, and tremors. The way Parkinson's manifests itself varies from person to person.

Though there is no total cure, life with Parkinson's can be made better. Through yoga, one can find a direction and discover techniques to manage Parkinson's symptoms. Yoga represents a non-medical form of treatment; it involves no drugs. The aims of yoga are physical flexibility (arthorosis prophylaxis), stress reduction (respiration), regulation of the cardiovascular system (decrease of hypertension), and an increase in physical energy (Pyhsical energy is produced in Mitochondria and measurable. A low level of bio-energy is an essential cause of numerous illnesses).

Yoga helps prevent Parkinson's, and it helps those who have it cope with and manage the disease. Yoga is one of the most ancient philosophical schools from Ancient India, a way of living which is 6000 years old. Yoga originates in the Indus Valley civilizations. The word "yoga" derives from the Sanskrit word "Yuj," which means "union," or "to connect." Therefore, it refers to the union of self-consciousness, or one person, with the universal consciousness. Yoga can be understood as a culture, science, psychology, art, form of spirituality, or simply as a way of living. What precisely yoga means depends on the individual practitioner and changes from person to person.

Swami Vivekananda, a Monk from India, first introduced Yoga to the West in 1893 at the World Parliament of Religions in Chicago. Since then, many Indian Monks and yoga teachers have taught yoga in the Western part of the world. Yoga practices have influenced many people, and they are often used as part of religion and body-mind medical systems throughout the world. Yoga exercises are also popular for reducing stress and improving flexibility.

Yoga is a critical tool for self-discovery. Modern science has given us so many technologies so that we can have a better quality of life. But with so much information and so many choices, it's increasingly easy for our senses to become overloaded. Our perception becomes confused, and our human intellect loses focus on discovering our true selves. Through the creation of systems and technological designs, chaos also emerges. Because of the analytical and rational neutrality of technology, it becomes more difficult to understand the abstract and conscious nature of human existence.

Yoga provides step-by-step guidance towards discovering the self. It starts from the physical bones and muscles, and with the increased connectivity between body and mind that it works towards, a yoga practitioner can learn to understand the complex mechanisms of the human body.

There are four directions for knowledge within yoga. But each direction contains a vast set of knowledge in itself. The four directions are:

1. Raja Yoga: Yoga of the mind; a controlled, scientific approach
2. Bhakti Yoga: Yoga of devotion; it involves prayer, music, and chanting for God
3. Karma Yoga: Path of the selfless service others
4. Gyana Yoga: Yoga of knowledge; it's an attempt at a philosophical and intellectual understanding of the world. It is sometimes also referred to as "jnana yoga."

In the following chapters, I will share the experiences of patients who underwent yoga therapy and Ayurvedic treatment. Afterwards, I will provide a guide to yoga and meditation practices that anyone with Parkinson's can use to ease their symptoms and increase their mindfulness.

ease their symptoms and increase their mindfulness.

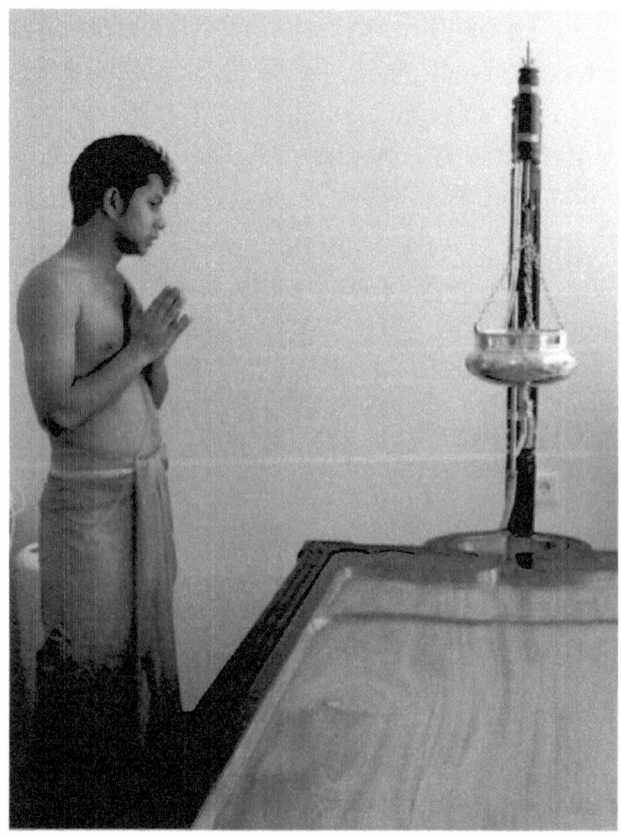

Dhroni,- A traditional Indian wooden Ayurvedic therapy bed from Kerala.

Chapter 3: Yoga Therapy and Ayurveda

The science of yoga begins to work on the outermost aspect of the personality, the physical body, which for most people is a practical and familiar starting point. When imbalances are experienced at this level, the organs, muscles, and nerves no longer function in harmony but are instead in tension with one another. For example, the endocrine system might become irregular, or the nervous system's efficiency might dwindle to such an extent that a disease manifests. Yoga aims to bring the different bodily functions into perfect coordination so that they work for the good of the whole body.

From the physical body, yoga moves on to operating at the mental and emotional levels. Many people suffer from phobias and neuroses as a result of the stresses in their lives. Yoga cannot provide a cure for these problems, but it does present a proven method for coping with it.

Each individual needs to find the form of yoga most suited to his/her particular personality and needs. In the last half of this century, hatha yoga has become the most well-known and widely practiced of the systems. However, the concept of what constitutes yoga is broadening as more people take up these practices.

Therapeutical Benefits of Hatha-Yoga

Research shows that yoga helps manage or control anxiety, arthritis, asthma, back pain, blood pressure, carpal tunnel syndrome, chronic fatigue, depression, diabetes, epilepsy, headaches, heart disease, multiple sclerosis, stress, and other conditions and dieases.

Practicing yoga has several beneficial effects:
- improves muscle tone, flexibility, strength, and stamina
- reduces stress and tension
- boosts self -esteem and confidence
- improves concentration, creativity, and coordination
- lowers fat and cholesterol
- improves circulation
- stimulates the immune system
- creates a sense of wellbeing and calm
- sets right psychosomatic disorders

General Benefits of Yoga: Physiological Benefits
- stable autonomic nervous system equilibrium with a tendency towards parasympathic nervous system dominance rather than the usual stress-induced sympathetic nervous system dominance
- Pulse rate decreases
- respiratory rate decreases
- blood pressure decreases (of special significance for hypo-reactors)
- galvanic skin response increases
- EEG alpha waves increase (theta, delta, and beta waves also increase during various stages of meditation)
- EMG activity decreases
- cardiovascular efficiency increases
- respiratory efficiency increases(respiratory
- amplitude and smoothness increase, tidal volume increases, vital capacity increases, and breath-holding time increases
- gastrointestinal function normalizes
- excretory function improves
- musculoskeletal flexibility and joint range of motion increase

- posture improves
- strength and resiliency increase
- endurance increases
- energy level increases
- weight normalizes
- sleep improves
- immunity increases
- pain decreases

Psychological Benefits of Yoga:
- somatic and kinesthetic awareness increase
- mood improves and subjective well being increase
- social adjustment increases
- anxiety and depression decreases
- hostility decreases
- psychomotor functions improve
- grip strength increases
- fine motor skill improves
- depth perception improves
- balance improves
- integrated functioning of the body parts improves
- cognitive function improves
- attention improves
- memory improves
- concentration improves
- symbol cording improves
- flicker fusion frequency improves

Biochemical Effects of Yoga:
- glucose decreases
- sodium decreases
- total cholesterol decreases
- triglycerides decreases
- HDL cholesterol increases

- LDL cholesterol decreases
- VDL cholesterol decreases
- cholinesterase increases
- catecholamine decreases
- ATPase increases
- haematocrit increases
- haemoglobin increases
- lymphocyte count increases
- total white blood cell count decreases
- thyroxin increases
- Vitamin C increases
- Total serum protein increases

Neurophysiological Effects of Yogic Practices

Scientists have shown that an experienced yogi can reduce his own metabolism and oxygen requirements. In a series of studies, minute auditory stimuli were given to subjects as they meditated, and their brain responses were recorded. Particular areas of the brain, particularly the thalamus, showed increased efficiency of activation. The breathing practices involved in yoga, *pranayama,* increases oxygen intake to the brain, which can help stimulate neurotransmitters. This creates more grey cells, thus improving the brain's health and functioning.

Raja Yoga for Parkinson's Patients

Raja yoga, or "royal yoga," is the path of systematic analysis and control of mind. Its steps were most notably compiled by Sage Patanjali Maharishi in the book called *Yoga Sutras.* In the two sub-paths of raja yoga, hatha yoga and kundalini yoga, the *prana* is mastered first, and the dormant kundalini energy is awakened. When we think of yoga in the West, we refer to only one of the eight limbs of raja yoga, namely hatha yoga, the practices of posture steadily held. Raja Yoga is also classically known as ashtanga yoga—"ashta" meaning "eight" and "anga" meaning "limb," as its practices can be divided into eight limbs. Raja yoga helps Parkinson's patients use systematic bodily analysis and control the mind and body with eight steps.

Step 1: *Yamas*—Self-regulation

a) *Ahimsa*—Non-violence and non-injury

In its true sense it means not to to desire to harm anybody with thoughts, words, or actions. This includes subtle forms of violence, such as speaking harshly or making clamorous sounds that may be injurious to others. It also means that you should not harm yourself by smoking, drinking alcohol, coffee, black tea, or getting depressed while dealing with Parkinson's. Treat your body as a temple; love and respect it.

b) *Satya*—Truthfulness

Truthfulness means not to lie under any circumstances. If you tell one lie, it will lead to others, which will not ever bring you peace of mind. Truthfulness is the way to happiness.

For those affected, it also means that you must face your Parkinson's. Accept that you have it, and don't try to hide it from yourself or others. That will help you reach peace with the disease.

c) *Asteya*—Avoidance of stealing

Refrain from taking what doesn't belong to you. If you have more than you need, then you are stealing from the rest of mankind. This also means that you shouldn't waste resources like water, electricity, or even take too long on the phone when others are waiting to use it. IAs Gandhi said, "There is enough in this world for everyone's need, but not for everyone's greed."

Do not steal your own health from yourself either. As you work towards recovery, don't deviate from your healthy practices. Find a balance in your activities in order to preserve your health and energy.

d) *Aparigraha*—Non-possessiveness

We always try to have more things than we use in our daily life, whether that's food, wealth, or physical space. As we struggle to maintain these standards, it robs us of happiness and peace of mind.

Although you should act with your health in mind, don't try to control your body or life. No control is the best control. Do not think obsessively about what will happen in the future; allow yourself to live in the moment.

e) *Brahmacharya*—Moderation

Moderation entails discipline of the senses. Its highest state is generally understood to be the transformation of sexuality to spirituality. It is sometimes misinterpreted as the suppression of sexual desire, which can lead to the suppression of other sensual activities.

Instead of suppression, all sensual pleasure should be enjoyed in moderation. Do not let eating, drinking, partying, or sex make you a slave to your senses.

Step 2: *Niyama*—Observations-

a) *Saucha*—Physical and mental cleanliness

Take a bath, give yourself a manicure, and put on perfumes to keep up your physical cleanliness. You should also keep up your mental wellbeing by following your ethics and morals to obtain personal happiness. Eliminate all distracting thoughts, and engage in meaningful conversation instead of small talk. Practice silence and punctuality in order to develop discipline of the mind.

b) *Santosha*—Contentment
   Very often, things happen that we didn't expected. Try to see both the sides of that situation, and see how the unexpected can be interpreted positively. *Santosha* helps us develop awareness, appreciation, and tolerance.

   Be content with your condition. Although Parkinson's is difficult, you don't have cancer or AIDS, nor were your hands or legs amputated. Try to think of the poor people suffering from more difficult diseases without anything to eat, drink, or wear in other parts of the world and close to home.

c) *Tapas*—Austerity and self-discipline
   Respecting your Parkinson's requires a lifestyle that involves activities such as doing exercises, taking medicine on time, going to bed regularly, and eating right.

d) *Swaadhyaaya*—Study of the self
   Write down your daily activities in a diary. Keep track of how you manage your movements and what you've learned. Through Parkinson's, you can find respect for your movements and for your life.

e) *Ishwarapranidhana*—Surrendering to God
   Stay on top of your Parkinson's treatments, and leave the rest to God. If you don't believe in God, then leave it to nature, luck, or your destiny.

   These practices help to purify the mind and eliminate its lower nature. If you are full of anger and greed, you cannot meditate well. This simple rule brings with it the more positive dimensions of life such as love, tolerance, and compassion.

Step 3: *Asanas*—Comfortable posture and movements

An *asana* is a posture in which the practitioner sits. Practicing *asanas* can improve your daily range of movements as well as your energy, stamina, motor functions, flexibility, balance, and physical coordination. It also helps to prevent the side effects of chemical medicines to some extent and to eliminate stress.

Step 4: *Pranayama*—Expansion of life energy

Yoga breathing techniques can help you manage tiredness, pain, and slow movement. It can also improve brain health by increasing the oxygen flow into brain cells. As it improves the body's life energy, it makes the immune system better.

Step 5: *Pratyahara*—Withdrawal of the senses

A turtle withdraws its body into its shell when it encounters an unpleasant touch. In the same way, we should withdraw our senses occasionally to avoid the unpleasantness of overindulgence. Withdrawing the senses helps improve non-motor symptoms like mood disorders and behavioral abnormalities. Yoga nidra, a state of consciousness between waking and sleeping, is a good technique for withdrawing the senses.

Step 6: *Dharana*—Concentration Practicing *dharana* helps increase the cognitive functions of the mind.

Step 7: *Dhyana*—Meditation-

Meditation is defined as an unbroken flow of thoughts towards Divinity to the exclusion of other sensual perceptions. When this concentration is maintained, unbroken, for about two minutes, one naturally falls into meditation. Then, there is no longer an awareness of space and time.

Meditation can bring peace to the soul, helping to separate you from the pain and sufferings of the body. It takes you to a special zone that exists outside of your body.

Step 8: *Samadhi*—-Super-conscious state
This refers to what is sublime beyond description: it's beyond the mind's ability to grasp. *Samadhi* transcends all ordinary, sensory experience as well as time, space and causation. *Samadhi* represents the goal of all existence. It is what all living beings are moving towards.

Samadhi, or the transcendental state, is also called *turiya,* the fourth state of consciousness. The three states of consciousness that we normally experience are waking, dreaming and dreamless sleep. When the mind reaches the point of concentration where meditation is maintained for about half an hour, it enters the fourth state in which the *upadhis*—limitations of body, senses, mind, and intellect--are transcended. Working towards *Samadhi* can help you reach the realization of a spiritual identity for your life with Parkinson's.

Bhakti Yoga for Parkinson's Patients
Bhakti yoga is the devotional approach to yoga, the approach of pure love. The *bhakta* (follower) does not try to rid himself of emotions, but instead seeks to channel and harness the emotions by sublimating them into devotion. The aspirant treading the path of bhakti attempts to realize the truth through devotion to and love of God in a personalized form. Prayer, chanting, *japa* (repeating a mantra or a name of God), hearing or telling stories of Gods and Saints, and ceremonies are all basic techniques of bhakti.

A mystical relationship with God(who may be seen as a friend, a child, a mother or teacher) is sought and developed through these practices. Bhakti yoga rids the aspirant of emotions and egocentricity by working towards humility, self-surrender and the feeling of being an instrument in the hands of God. Ideally, the bhakti yogi finds the presence of God in the heart's center, and when they do so, their whole life is experienced as a visceral oneness with the divine.

Bhakti yoga can help Parkinson's patients improve speech control and reduce depression. Singing loudly with emotion and rhythm can also help Parkinson's patients improve their speech ability. Freestyle dancing can help with improving motor functions and concentration as well as reducing depression. Devotional chants, prayer, and music are essential to bhakti yoga. I recommend listening to Krishna Das, Jai Uttal, or Deva Premal.

Karma Yoga for Parkinson's Patients

Karma yoga is the yoga of self-transcending action. Mahatma Ghandhi is perhaps the most well-known of recent karma yogis. In karma yoga, we act upon the world and all beings in the spirit of transcendent selfless service. One lives life with a recognition of the divine in all things. The Indian greeting "Namaste" explains the idea behind this practice well; it means "The divine in me recognizes the divine in you."

Karma yoga involves the dedication of all work as an offering to God, with no thought of personal reward. A karma yogi attempts to see the Lord dwelling in all living beings. By renouncing the fruits of one's action, the action becomes unselfish. By not thinking of our own personnel needs and desires and trying to help everybody around us (including human beings, animals, and the planet) the heart is expanded, egoism is destroyed, and one-ness is realized. Karma yoga can be practiced at all times under all conditions; it is applicable anywhere there is a desire to do selfless service. One resource for better understanding karma yoga is the *Bhagavat Gita*.

Karma yoga can help Parkinson's patients work and move without stress. It teaches how to live in the moment without thinking about the past or the future. Yoga is not so much about intelligence; it is about awareness, a creative response to the present. Using intelligence to assess which movements are good or bad brings stress, and with the mind, a patient may linger on memories of being fit and healthy as well as fear of the future. Instead, you should be aware of the present; just focus on *now*.

Gyana Yoga for Parkinson's Patients

Gyana yoga is the yoga of wisdom. Through philosophical study, dialogue and debate, the gyana yogi aspires to the ideal of non-dualism, in which reality is seen as singular and distinct from the perception that we are separate from the divine. This illusory concept of separation is referred to as *Maya*. Sri Sankaracharya stands as the spokesman of gyana yoga and proclaims that "The universe is unreal; only Bhrama is real." All things that are subject to change are unreal. It is only the unchanging that is real.

Through the study of Vedanta philosophy, the gyani tries to learn to discriminate between what is finite (and therefore unreal) and the infinite. Dispassion (*vairagya*) is then developed. Vedanta maintains that liberation cannot be attained by ritual, action, duty or charity; it can only be reached through personal intuitive experience.

Vedanta philosophy is based in scripture, reason, and experience, but it does not demand blind faith. While Vedantins take the scriptures as authority, they must analyze and understand all the teachings using their own intellect. After exhausting, through the process of discrimination and negation, all that is unreal, the intellect too must be discarded. Only the experience of the real remains. This is self-realization.

Gyana yoga is the most direct of the four paths. It is the intellectual approach to spiritual evolution. Through the right inquiry (*vichara*) and constant self –analysis (*viveka*) the mind is used to examine its own nature. However, gyana yoga is said to be the most difficult path, not because it is superior but because one must be firmly grounded in the other disciplines before attempting it. A sharp, keen intellect, unclouded by emotions, is necessary.

Gyana yoga can help Parkinson's patients better understand their own lives. It can help bring about the realization that there is nothing permanent or secure, not even for the doctors, therapists, and nurses who treat a patients. A healthy man without Parkinson's may die from any of a number of sudden causes before a Parkinson's patient.

Ayurveda--- Complementary Medicine- Ayurveda-Traditional Indian Medicine-

Kampa Vata is the name of Parkinson in Ayurveda for 4500 years.It is said in bengali language "Bhuri bhalo to Muri Bhalo".That means if digestion and elimination is proper then your brain functioning is also proper. Ayurveda says Constipation is the mother of all Diseases.So the diseases start from intestines.

Also in modern research in Germany it agrees that Parkinson's starts in Intestine 12 years before it manifests in Physical body.

Mucuna pruriens is a plant of the legume family that has been used by Ayurvedic Practitioners to treat Parkinson's for more than 4,500 years; western medicine is now accepting mucuna as an alternative treatment to, or complementary therapy with,L-dopa, as a study after study is proving its effectiveness. Research cited by the National Parkinson Foundation found that " dose to dose,mucuna was two to three times more effective than equivalent amounts of Synthetic drugs." The Ayurvedic Internal Medicines,Ayurvedic massages and specially the Ayurvedic Detoxification program for 14 to 21 days known as Panchakarma can really help Parkinson patients. After an Ayurvedic Thearapy Program for 3 or 4 weeks Parkinson pateints feel better, quality of movements and life also improves.

Ayurveda is a Traditional Indian Medicine (TIM) originating from Indian Culture.

Ayur means life and Veda means knowledge, Ayurveda means Knowledge of Life.

Parkinson and Yoga

Yoga represents a non – medical form of treatment without any chemical drugs for humans. Aim of Yoga is Physical flexibility(arthrosis prophylaxis),stress reduction(respiration),regulation of the cardiovascular system(decrease of Hypertension), increase of Physical energy(Pyhsical energy is produced in Mitochondria and measurable. A low level of bio-energy is an essential cause of numerous illnesses).

So in short Parkinson Yoga can manage & improve the quality of life of patients by suggesting-

1. Proper eating concept(Sattwic Ahar)
2. Proper Expression of body and soul(Chanting,Singing Bhajans,LaughingYoga,Face Yoga,Yoga Dancing)
3. Proper Energy intake and Use(Pranayama,Prathayahara,Sharir Dharana)
4. Proper Quality Movements in daily life.(Asanas)

Parkinson and Ayurveda

Scope of Ayurveda in this book is very limited. As Traditionally Ayurvedic approach of Treatment is very individualistic. An Ayurvedic Doctor in India will not classify the Parkinson patient as a patient but an individual and try to balance Vata and its Avaranas.

With special Ayurvedic protocals like

1. Internal medicines ---Kasayam,Curnam,bhasma,tailam,aristam,etc,
2. External physical therapies ----Udvartanam,Thalam,Abhyangam,etc

3. Detoxification -----Nasyam,Vasti,Virecanam,etc

Ayurveda is a other world in itself- One needs a proper setup, special therapies beds,equipments, Properly Trained Ayurveda Therapist and overall a Properly Educated Ayurvedic Doctor who can really understand and apply the principles according to the need of the patients.

Now days Ayurveda or Wellness Ayurveda is very popular, Every big hotel offer Realxing ayurvedic massages and getting a Proper Medical Ayurvedic Setup is Difficult.

So patients have to be very careful in selecting a place and an Ayurvedic Doctor.

And most important the patient should be interested and open for the world of Ayurveda. Specially for the Diet, Lifestyle and be ready to invest Time and Money.

Generally an Ayurvedic Program lasts for 14 to 21 days, sometimes even more days are required. A patient has to stay in the Ayurvedic Clinic and follow certain preparation before and ending routine after the Ayurvedic Program.

What one can take from this book is the Ayurvedic Daily routine, that I write in the next chapter. That one can easily follow.

You can ask your doctor whether you can try Mucuna pruriens as a natural subsititute for L-dopa intake.

This simple daily routine from Ayurveda and the Yoga Movements can help a lot in the process of healing.

Mucuna pruriens is a plant of the legume family that has been used by Ayurvedic Practitioners to treat Parkinson's.

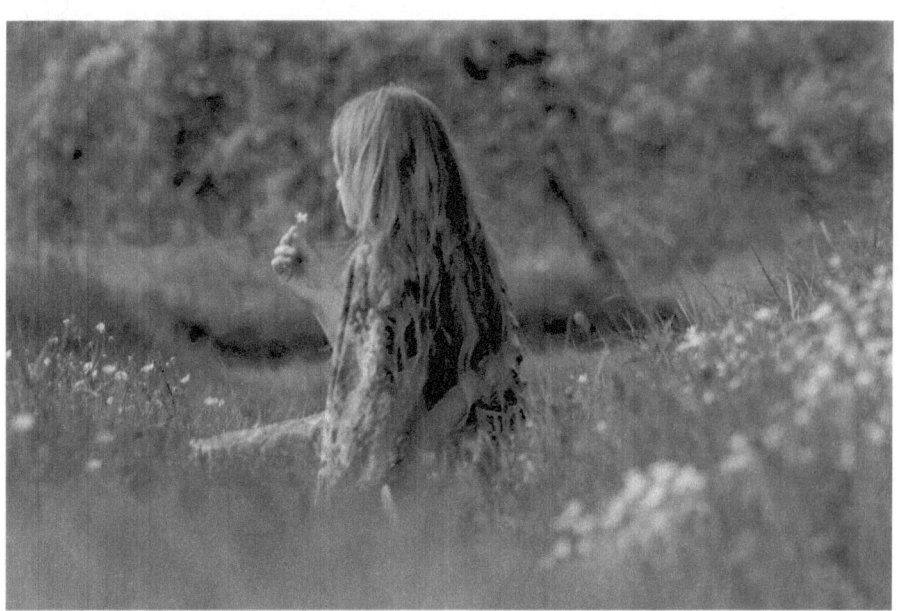

Chapter 4: Yoga and the Ayurvedic Lifestyle for Parkinson's Patients

The yoga lifestyle is not a set of rules; instead, it is a body of knowledge built on thousands of years of experience, meant to help you find your way to health.

Yoga therapy is based on four principles:

1. *Dahuti*—Detoxification
2. *Asana*—Psychophysical somatic movements
3. *Pranayama*—Breathing techniques to improve life energy
4. *Dhyana*—Mindfulness with meditative awareness

For Parkinson's patients, however, these principles can be modified and reconsidered as follows:

1. *Sattwic Ahar*—Proper eating
2. Proper expression of the body and soul (chanting, singing, laughing, yoga, and dance)
3. Proper energy intake and use *(Pranayama, Prathayahara,* and *Sharir Dharana)*
4. Proper quality of movements and daily meditation *(Asanas, Vedanta* and *Dhyana)*

Yogic Lifestyle for Parkinson's Patients

1) Proper eating

According to the concept of *sattwic ahar,* or the yogic diet, food serves as the basis of the body, mind, and soul. Eating right gives balance and harmony to the body.

The yogic diet is based on pure food, which is grown or created naturally rather than a hybrid product of biotechnology. Master yogis eat only ripe fruits and water, but for most people the diet also includes nuts, vegetables, fruits, cereals, honey, and milk. It excludes eggs, flesh, and fish because these don't give as much energy, as they come from products lower on the food chain. One can find all the essential nutrients (proteins, fats, carbohydrates, and minerals) in a vegetarian diet.

Modern medicines for Parkinson's patients, including those that use the amino acid, L-dopa cannot function properly when you take animal protein. Protein from vegetables actually works better in conjunction with modern medicine.

It's also best to avoid milk products, as they create mucus in the intestines. Parkinson's patients in particular should be concerned with the health of their intestines and digestive system.

Exciting and overly-stimulating things like coffee, black tea, cigarettes, alcohol, and excessive sex should also be avoided, as they stress the nervous system. Since Parkinson's weakens the nervous system, it's important not to damage it in other ways.

Some Parkinson's patients think that it's impossible to eat without consuming any kind of animal flesh, but in our neurological ward, patients stay for eighteen days and subsist of a diet without bread, coffee, animal flesh, eggs, fish, or alcohol. Most of our patients follow this diet successfully — and these are Germans learning to manage without their bread and coffee!

This diet also helps people who are overweight reach a healthy body weight, and it helps underweight patients improve their digestive power through their breathing and movements.

When you are sick, food isn't fun; it's a medicine. Bread, Meat and processed foods creates constipation and hard for the intestines to digest. Please Focus on your health, not your taste buds only.

Some basic guidelines for a Parkinson's diet:

1. Please drink lukewarm water and Avoid refrigerated water, wine, coffee, or black tea; in the long run, these drinks all make your nervous system weak. You can experiment with new drinks like herbal tea or ginger tea. As a treat, enjoy hot chocolate without whipped cream sometimes.

2. Generally bread and cheese are hard to digest. Instead, enjoy porridge, oats, and fresh fruit salads.

3. Instead of non-vegetarian proteins like meat, fish, and eggs, consume proteins through nuts, spinach, and beans. These will work better in conjunction with modern Parkinson's medicine. If you're really struggling with not eating meat, you can consume bird meat (chicken, turkey, or duck) as they are easier to digest than beef or pork. Fish causes mucus in the body and slows movement, so it's best to avoid fish as well.

4. Avoid milk products like cheese, butter, and ice cream—milk products create mucus in the body. Instead, consume coconut milk or soy milk, and use olive oil or other plant-based cooking oil.

5. Always eat cooked, boiled, or otherwise warm food. Salads are raw and cold, which makes them harder to digest. If you need to eat salads, yogurts, or other raw foods, it's best to eat them in the morning; this is when your digestive power is strongest.

6. Eating is like meditation. Eat quietly, and chew many times before swallowing. Don't attempt to multitask while eating. Turn off your phone or television, and avoid lunch meetings. Don't stress your brain, body, and nerves by trying to do too many things at the same time.

2) Proper Expression of body and soul

As a patient with Parkinson's, it's important to remember that existence is based in expression and awareness. Think about driving a car, for example; it doesn't require intelligence or even concentration, but as you drive, you aware of your own connectivity to the car. You consider its turning radius, the space it takes to park, how much room you need to stop before a red light. Your existence is connected to the car's; this is what awareness truly means.

As a Parkinson's patient, you can use yoga as a way to develop and channel mindfulness. Even with motor disabilities, laughing yoga, dance yoga, and chair yoga are all options that are available to you.

3) Proper energy intake and use

It's also important to remember to intake and use energy properly. Growing older means no longer having the intense energy of a teenager; likewise, when suffering from a disease, the body naturally has less energy. It's therefore necessary to conserve it for the best possible use. Most people don't think about the energy that it takes to speak, walk, or make facial expressions, but when a patient has Parkinson's, these tasks no longer seem so simple. You must relearn how to use your body in a new way. As with carrying a child, you must allow your movements to adjust; now, your body is like the body of the child.

One tool for doing this is *pranayama,* yogic breathing. Oxygen gives us energy, so yogic breathing is essentially the expansion of life energy. *Pranayama* brings balance and harmony to both the physical body and to the mind. Most of us don't use our full lung capacity. All classic yogic breathing techniques are based on proper diaphragm movements so as to use our lungs as fully as possible.

For the diaphragm to move evenly, the spine must be straight, so improving breathing aids posture as well. The increased oxygen intake also improves blood quality and helps the nervous system, relaxing the muscles and bones.

As oxygen flow to the brain increases, the grey cell count increases. By changing the electrical wave pattern in the brain, one can harmonize the left and right brain hemispheres. In addition to improving body movement, this contributes to the development of self-confidence and stress reduction.

It's also important to practice *pratyahara,* or yogic relaxation. Relaxation allows us to recharge our brain, senses, and cognitive powers. The body and mind become tired, and we withdraw ourselves and our senses in order to recharge.

Yoga nidra, a technique from the Bihar School of Yoga, is a good technique for *pratyahara.* When done correctly, it can help you find self-confidence and strength within yourself.

Sarir Dharana

Another aspect of Ayurvedic treatment is *sarir dharana,* stability of bodily functions. But the body is always changing as it seeks homeostasis; how can you find stability in such a situation?

For Parkinson's patients, it's best to think of *sarir dharana* as a kind of bodily awareness that comes after practice of *pranayama* and *pratyahara.* It's an understand and realization that finding stability takes time. It functions as a middle way, a path of balance between health and illness.

4) Proper quality movemnets and daily meditation.

When considering the importance of proper bodily movements and meditation, most people think of *asanas,* yogic movement. But you should not just think of the exterior body; *asanas* require the cooperation of the brain, heart, muscles, nerves, and endocrine system in order to find a state of harmony and balance.

Become aware of the way your body exists with Parkinson's. Don't judge yourself based on perceived health or sickness. Instead, think about why you are using different yoga movements and postures, and be satisfied with your own movements. Don't criticize your hands for shaking or your legs for staggering. Simply be aware of the way your body functions, and allow yourself to experience your own movements.

The Indian school of *Vedanta* claims that every human is the master of his/her own life, a philosophy that can be useful for those living with Parkinson's. Remember not to judge your own situation but instead work on moving forward. The greatest sin in life, it suggests, is to think that you are weak.

Vedanta philosophy can motivate Parkinson's patients to become the masters of their own lives. It claims that self-help is the best help; it's important to find the power within yourself. You must become your own healer. Try different medicines, and focus on developing the sources of your own strength.

Vedanta teaches that you should live every moment of your life fully, and accept that life is perpetual movement forward. Life consists of movement. Even on days where you feel tired, stiff, and dizzy, try not to label is as "feeling good" or "feeling bad." Simply allow yourself to live, and focus on moving forward.

One way of living in the moment is *dhyana,* yogic meditation. *Dhyana* is not concentration; instead, it refers to a form of becoming. Think of a baby, always falling and putting new things into its mouth—babies are perpetually curious and experiencing life. They are like yogis, but without self-awareness.

For someone with Parkinson's, yogic meditation requires moving with and becoming one with Parkinson's, just as a man or woman does with a spouse.

Detoxification (Shatkarma & Panchakarma) Yoga therapy start with this. But yoga detoxification are very physical and strenuous – a yogic technique- laghoo sankhaprakshalana(cleaning the entire gastro intestinal track) will be useful for Parkinson patients. But it is very difficult to perform. If the patient is in early stages then he can try to do it once every month. But Parkinson patients can be better handled with Ayurvedic Detoxification- Known as Panchakarma. Always consult a doctor before trying this detoxification process.

So a Parkinson patient with a proper eating concept(sattwic Ahar)-detoxifies his body, helping the body and digestive function to work easily. As it takes long time to digest flesh foods that are also acid in nature and warm cooked food is always easy to digest too. With proper expression of body and soul one can manage depression and can achieve quality movements and facial expressions. Life energy management is an important aspect of healing and through detoxification life energy prana can flow freely.

Parkinson disease as with this complex neurological problem one does not have enough natural life force.The breathing exercises Pranayama and Prathayahara will improve the cognitive and perception abilities.and Sharir dharana will give an integration effect to the body, mind and soul. Proper quality movements like asanas will give an somatic experience by reducing the muscle tone and improving the motor function by balancing the nervous system. Vedanta philosophy will give motivation and by doing Dhyana one can attain peace. So with the help of Yogic lifestyle one can manage Parkinson and improve the quality of life with better movements, expressions and mental satisfaction.

And Ayurvedic lifestyle with help to balance life energy and organ functions by removing the toxins with the Detoxification known as Panchakarma. I recommend every year or every two year if a Parkinson patient does the Ayurveda panchakarma, the life quality will be better.

Ayurvedic Routine

Here is a suggested daily Ayurvedic routine that most Parkinson's patients can do at home.

Morning Plan
- Rise early, between 5:30 and 5:45 am.
- Wash your face and mouth with water.
- Scrape your tongue with a tongue scraper to clean the white coating.
- Use 20 ml of sesame oil or another cooking oil to gargle and clean your mouth.
- Drink one cup of warm water after it's been boiled, and go to the toilet.
- Take one spoonful of coconut oil, and then drink one cup of warm water with a teaspoonful of lemon juice.
- Dip your index finger in the cooking oil, bring it to your nostrils, and inhale deeply. Let the oil stay there for five to ten minutes before wiping your nose with tissue paper.
- Give your head, hands, and feet a massage with the sesame oil.
- Take a bath in warm water.
- Practice yoga 1 and 2, followed by breathing exercises and meditation.

Eating Plan

- Have breakfast early. Eat porridge, oats, boiled rice, or boiled fruits and vegetables. Avoid bread, black tea, and coffee. Don't consume raw, cold food like salads.
- Enjoy a vegetarian or vegan lunch sometime between noon and 2:00 pm.
- After lunch, try to take a short walk in a park or garden, or enjoy a silent pause on your porch or balcony.
- Between 3:00 pm and 5:00 pm, enjoy herbal tea or another healthy snack.
- Eat a light, warm dinner such as a vegan or vegetarian soup. Eat dinner early, and avoid raw salads, cheese, and yogurt at night.
- After 8:00 pm, relax and prepare to sleep.

Sleeping Plan

- Before bed, give yourself a foot massage with a cream or oil
- Listen to instrumental music. It's typically best to enjoy something light, like flutes or string instruments.
- Go to bed early in order to sleep well.

Some of my patients improved during their twenty-one day stays at the hospital, but after they left, they returned to their old eating and living habits. Of course, when they did so, their symptoms began to manifest.

Patients sometimes invited me to their home for yoga therapy, and when they do so, I'll ask about their eating habits and lifestyles. I'm sometimes invited to eat ice cream or drink wine with my Parkinson's patients, which is uncomfortable, but I don't want to insult them by refusing. When I'm a guest, I cannot also be a strict Ayurvedic therapist and yoga teacher.

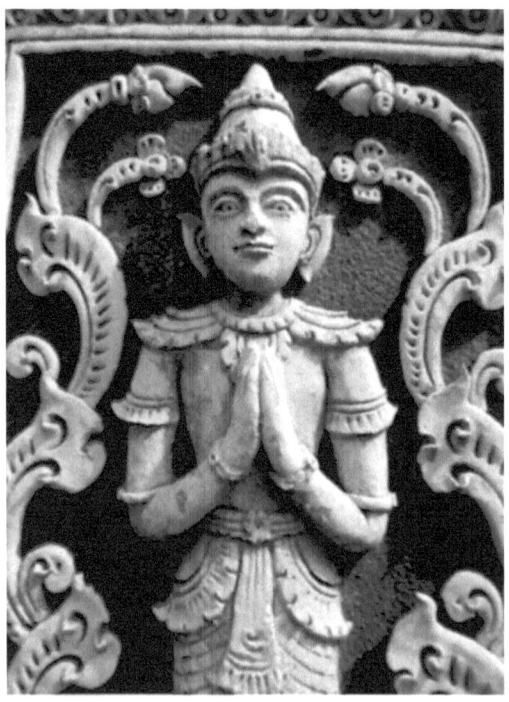

PART 2 –
MANAGEMENT

Manage what you can in the present rather than focusing on the past or future. If you manage the present, then the past and future will find balance as well.

Chapter 5: Self-Confidence

A baby is a born leader. It has incredible self-confidence. It doesn't hesitate to move, and it never asks permission to do anything; it just does, and others follow. But unlike babies, we as adults can develop goals.

Nature too is independent. It doesn't require the help of mankind, and even after natural disasters, it heals itself, returning to balance and harmony. Human civilizations have been around for thousands of years, but nature predates society.

A yogic lifestyle works towards bringing about harmony and balance in your bodily systems, which helps build self-confidence. Yoga teaches you to become an individual who works to better yourself, not necessarily to become a perfectly productive social individual.

In a spiritual sense, yoga is about creating a connection with the ever-changing present. The body is never static; every day, old cells are dying and new ones are born. If your body was perfect, it would be a stone statue in a museum.

Consider the world-famous scientist Stephen Hawking. Many people might consider him handicapped because he sits in a wheelchair and cannot speak normally. If Hawking thought about his disease this way, it would have been easy for him to become depressed. However, he has connected to the wheelchair and computer to communicate, interacting with the present the way most people would with their body parts. Although I don't know him personally, I find him highly inspirational.

Find self-confidence in yoga through using the diaphragm to fill your muscles, bones, and organs with life energy. Use steady poses to develop confident body language. Yogic relaxation, *pratyahara*, helps you develop a better understanding of the body's consciousness and awareness by providing self-perception and improved cognition. Additionally, a yogic diet improves your energy, compassion, and kindness, as you're helping the environment and world at large through your eating habits.

Through these practices, you can find the energy and self-confidence that will not only help with healing but will help you enjoy your existence.

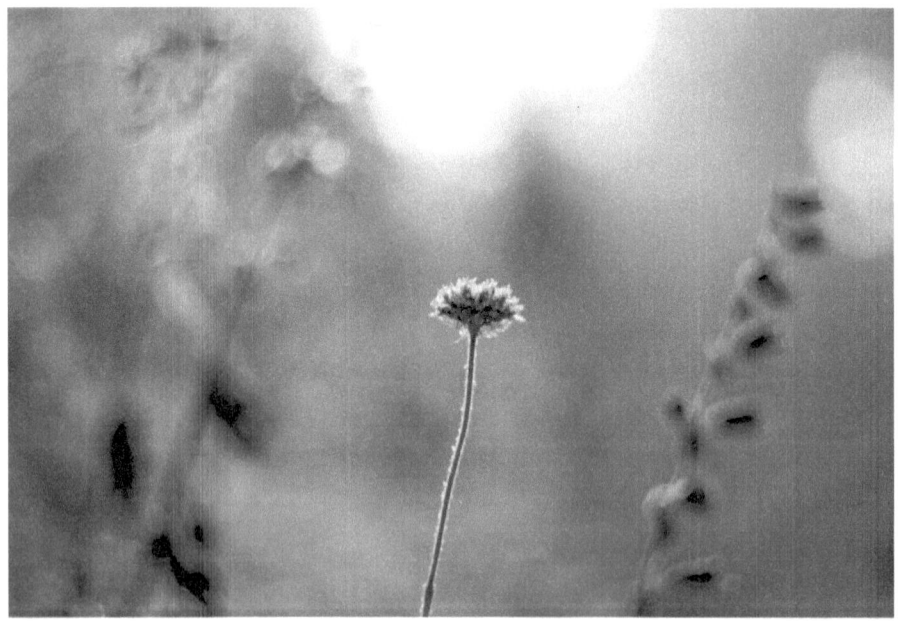

Chapter 6: Spirituality

The ultimate aim of yoga is to find peace within, and in this regard, yoga is a spiritual science. Although Yoga is a Indian philosophy, it espouses universal spiritual elements from which all people can benefit in order to find peace, harmony, and balance.

One yogic tool for spirituality is the *mantra,* which means a sound encased in energy that frees one from the mind. Sometimes, the mind is so cluttered that it becomes difficult to focus, which in turn gives way to stress, tension, burnout, or more serious psychological problems.

Suppose you're sitting in a chaotic place, and you hear a sound that calmly, repetitively cuts through the chaos. Your mind will focus on this sound, and your attention will be directed towards it automatically. This is how a *mantra* works; chanting a mantra cut through the chaos of the mind. Once you are able to create focus, you'll find quietness and peace.

AUM is the most popular *mantra.* It is a Sanskrit word, and it is believed that this represents the first vibrating sound which created the world. In this way, it represents the absolute. It has been used by millions of worshippers and has become so universal that it refers to no deity in particular.

Swami Vivekananda said that the first letter, A, creates the root sound, pronounced without touching any part of the tongue or palate. The final M represents the last sound, as it's produced with a closed lip. The U rolls from the very root to the ending sound, so AUM represents the phenomena of sound production.

From a therapeutic perspective, this *mantra* requires harmony of the lungs, diaphragm, abdomen, throat, tongue, nose, and lips.

Repeating it massages the inner organs through vibration, therefore improving cognition and relaxing the nervous system. Chanting properly requires breathing from the diaphragm, which in turn allows the brain to receive more oxygen.

There are several Sanskrit hymns that one can use when practicing yoga or meditation. -Sanskrit is one of the oldest Indo-European languages, and many words in other European languages derive from Sanskrit. These hymns are from the *Vedas,* one of the oldest books in the world, but their meanings are still universally applicable.

It's common to chant hymns at the beginning and end of yoga and meditation, but they can be used any time one seeks mental peace.

Below is the translation of one Sanskrit *mantra:*

SHANTI MANTRA

AUM SAHA NAVAVATU
SAHA NAU BHUNAKTU
SAHA VIRYAM KARAVAAHAI
TEJASVI NAVADHITAMASTU
MA VIDVISHAVAHAI
AUM SHANTI SHANTI SHANTI

The meaning in English is as follows:

Hymn for Peace

Protect us together
Nourish us together
Put our efforts together
There should not be any ill will or bad thoughts
Let our knowledge illuminate
We should not quarrel with each other
Peace be, peace be, peace be

Note that the idea of peace first refers to peace for the personal body, mind, and soul. Second, it addresses peace for all living and non-living things on Earth. Finally, it asks for universal peace for all that is known and that which is still unknown.

SHANTI PATH

ASATO MA SADGAMAYA
TAMASO MA JYOTIRGAMAYA
MRITYORMA AMRITAM GAMAYA
AUM SHANTI SHANTI SHANTI

Prayer for peace

Lead me from untruth to truth
Lead me from darkness to light
Lead me from death and disease to Moksha (mortality to immortality)
peace be, peace be, peace be

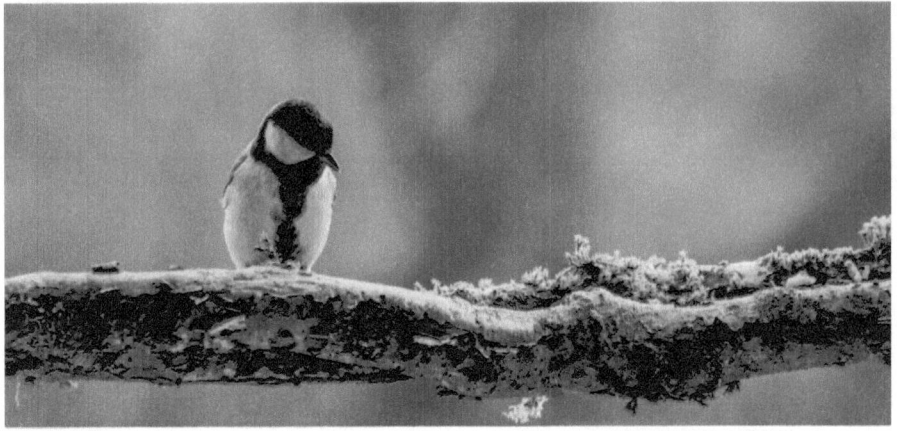

Chapter 7: Parkinson's Yoga

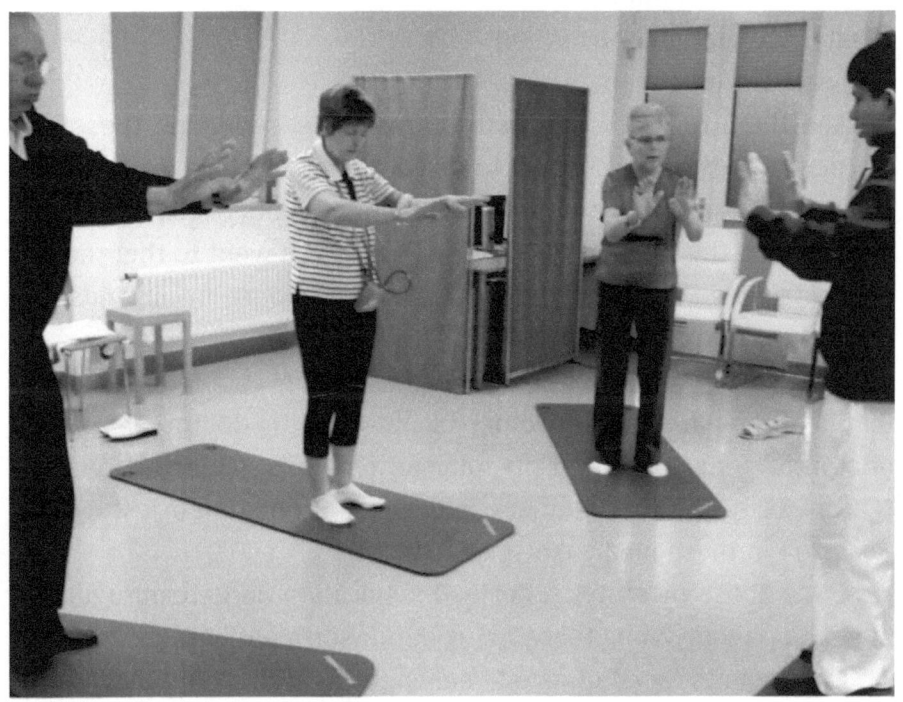

When Professor Horst Przuntek invited me to develop a Parkinson's yoga program in Germany, I knew little about the disease other than that Mohammed Ali had Parkinson's.

A very personal experience from my childhood was that my mother used to motivate a Parkinson patient who was my neighbor to move and walk and as a childs play I used to take steps with him was also helpful for me.

I arrived at the hospital to teach my first one-hour yoga class knowing only three German words and I had ten patients standing in front of me. I have to speak in German and I do not know how to take a class for one hour in german language.

I pointed to my nose, took a deep breath, and asked how to say "inhalation" in German. One kind German Patient said-*Einatmen.*

I repeated – Einatmen.
What is Exhalation? *Ausatmen.*
I repeated - Ausatmen
I asked them to follow my body movements, repeating these two German words in succession to direct their breathing. My patients learned by watching, and I watched the patients. I observed their movements, their gestures, and over time even went to their homes and befriended many of them. The patients were my friends, my philosophers, and my guides.

Every week once we had a team meeting about the developments of the patients. Neurologists, naturopathy doctors, Ayurveda doctors, nurses, psychiatrists, physiotherapists, speech and dance therapists, health practitioners, and even a Protestant priest used to take part in these medical discussions.

From these meetings, I derived inspiration and encouragement in developing my yoga therapy for Parkinson's patients.

My patients faced unusual challenges as well. Many had fluctuating blood pressure or brain stimulators. Some relied on walkers and wheelchairs, and others had little cognitive power left. Some of these patients battled challenges like MS or chronic depression.

I taught two yoga classes each day. The first, Yoga I, was for mobile patients who had normal motor functions. The second was for immobile patients, and most of those in my Yoga II class used sticks, walkers, or wheelchairs for most of their daily activities. For this second group of patients, my main challenge was to alter yoga movement techniques according to each person's specific needs.

Here were the rules I asked my students to follow:
1. **Move before you understand why.**
   First move, and then understand. When you move, your nerve impulses send messages to brain, and your autonomic nervous system tries to reach homeostasis. Somatic movements (*asanas*) interact with and improve your cognitive state (*chetana*). Bodily awareness is different from intelligence. If needed close your eyes while practicing yoga in order to relax the brain and nervous system and improve your self-perception.
2. **Do not label movements as "good" or "bad."**
   Movement is living. Move without thinking of the result, or you'll bring about stress and depression that will only worsen your symptoms and prevent your wellbeing.
3. **No control is the best control**
   We like to think we can control our own bodies, but the body has its own wisdom and forms of knowledge. When you practice yoga, don't concentrate on controlling your movements; just focus on love.
4. **Perfection is a stupid concept.**
   A computer is perfect, but it lacks creativity. A work of art may be perfect, but then it is static and unchanging. Don't judge your wellbeing by the movements you made before Parkinson's. Try to find harmony in the chaos.

With these guidelines in mind, I have provided yoga routines for those with Parkinson's. Try following these suggestions and experiencing the sensation of movement.

Do not label movements as "good" or "bad."

Yoga for the Mobile Patient (YOGA I)

Balance, Coordination, and Breathing

Come into a standing posture, feel the contact of your foot's sole with your mat. Lift the toes up (fig.1). Contract your knee caps. Push your chest out, and you're your head high.

Now, put your toes down, and feel the center of your body. Grip the mat with your toes and play with the weight of your body. Shift forward and backward, forward and backward.

Now, move from side to side, left and right. Slowly, return your body to the center. Try to find balance and grounding by keeping your spine, neck, and head straight. Please repeat this 5 to 10 times and find the easy way.

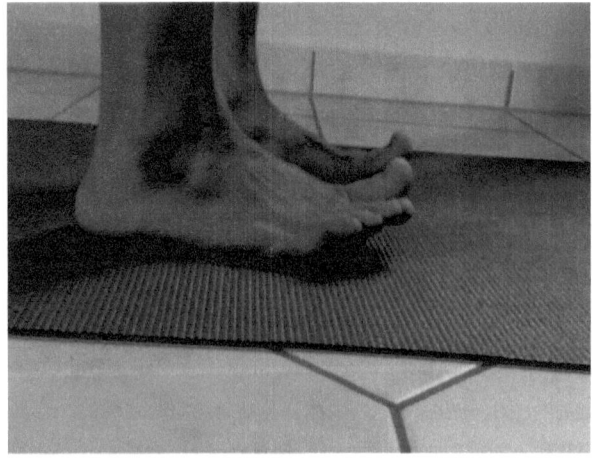

Figure 1

Now keep the right hand on the naval and left hand on the middle of the chest (fig.2). Practice abdominal breathing; as you inhale the abdomen comes out. As you exhale, the abdomen goes in towards the spine. Inhale. The abdomen comes out. Exhale. The abdomen goes in towards the spine. Keep doing this, using the full capacity of your lungs. Ground yourself in this bodily alignment. Whenever you stand, try to maintain this alignment. Again, inhale and exhale, and feel your abdomen's movement. Slowly return to a normal standing position and drop your hands to your sides. One can use this breathing while freezings states.Practice this for 2 to 5 minutes as you feel comfortable. While practicing feel how to abdomen muscles and back muscles react to your breathing, how the breathing supports your balance, posture and movement.

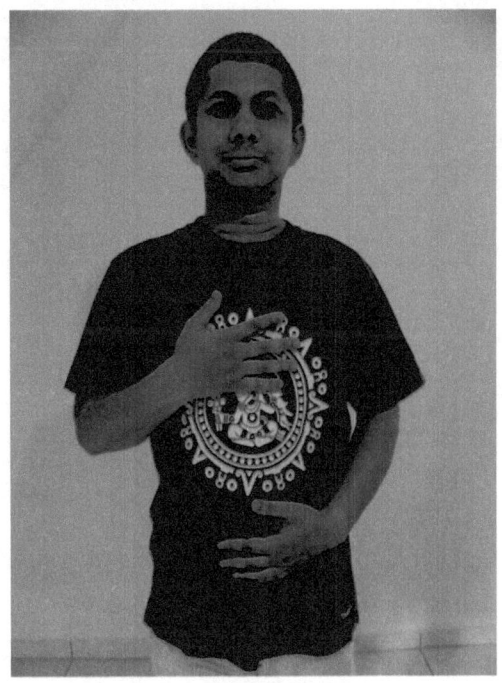

Figure 2

Now keep your hands under your naval. As you inhale, lift your hands up as much as you can (fig 3). As you exhale, bend your knees and bring your hands to your knees (fig. 4). Repeat this pattern of breathing and movement without stressing your muscles or joints. As you do this, feel your body's coordination. When you move, turn or walk; you need the coordination of arms and legs. Feel the opening of ribcage, especially the small muscles in between the ribcage. Repeat this five to ten times, try to inhale and exhale through nose only, not through mouth. Try to keep the brain soft, then one can easily exhale through nose, Exhaling through the mouth does not allow your organs to get the best of oxygen intake from the normal air.

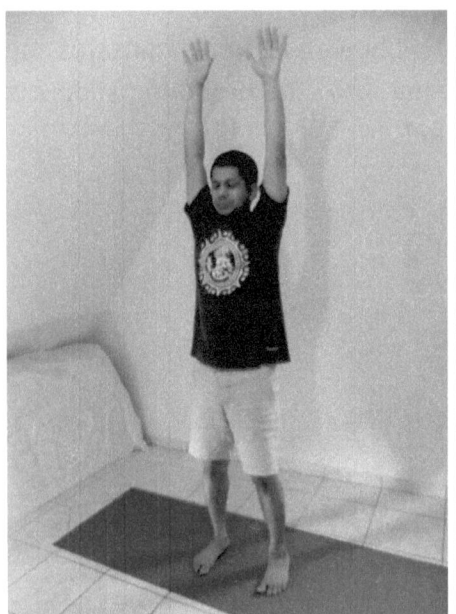 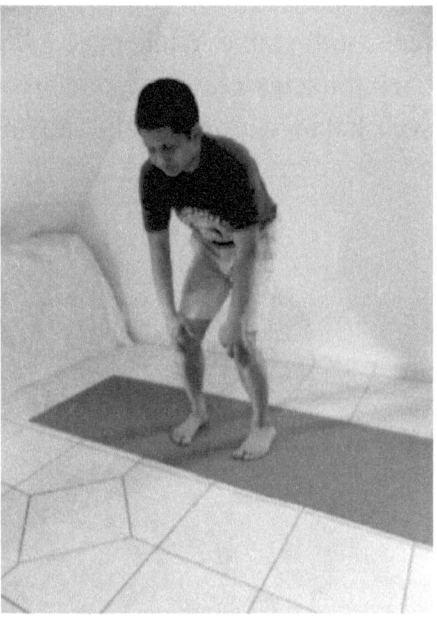

Figure 3   Figure 4

Slowly come into a standing posture. With your right hand, use the index finger and thumb to grab your left ear, and use the fingers of your left hand to do the same to your right ear (fig.5). Inhale, and slowly bend your knees into a sitting position as much as you can (fig.6). And as you exhale, come into the standing posture. Again, inhale as you sit down, and exhale as you come up. Repeat these movements, allowing the stress to leave your body. Afterwards, return to a standing position and put your hands at your sides.

This movement may look strange, by pulling the ears, you are relaxing the brain, making it soft, and trying to feel the fluids in the ear, responsible for your sense of balance. By bending the knees and crossing the arms one can understand the joint spaces and angles in movement. So in daily life when more complex situation comes with movement, one can use this practice and understanding to manage that situation.

Practice this for five or Ten times as you feel comfortable.

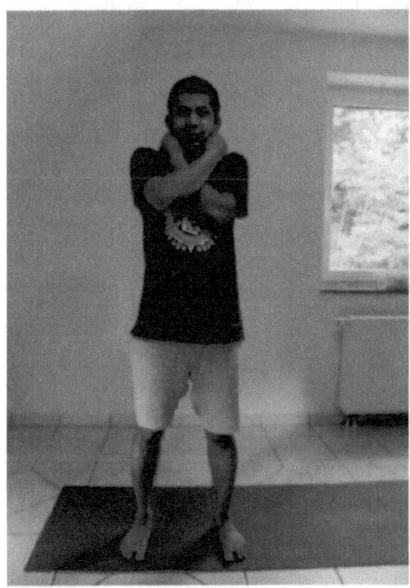 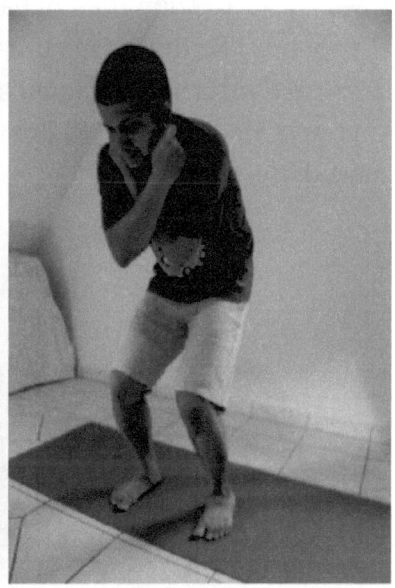

Figure 5 Figure 6

Next, place both hands on your head, one on top of the other (fig.7). Press down just enough to feel a small amount of pressure in your throat. Inhale and exhale through your nose, and feel these movements in your throat. Now, with each inhalation, try to feel your spine. As you exhale, relax the spine, throat, and nostrils. Feel these breaths as they pass through you.

Head is the heaviest part of the body, if one can feel the weight of the head and connection to the legs, keeping balance is possible without much muscular effort, then new ways to connect with the brain and gravity can be learned.Breath has direct connection with nervous function,oxygen can cross the blood brain region naturally and can give a new connection with the body and mind. Practice this for 2 to 5 minutes, one can also sit in a chair and even lie on the back and practice this yoga breathing.

Do not overstrain the throat, try to listen to the sound of breath, in yoga world its is known as oceanic breath, as the sounds of your breath sounds like the waves breaking on the beach and going away. In Classical Sanskrit it is known as Ujjayi Pranayama, Think you are sucking and pulling fruit juice with the help of a straw but the lips are closed and relaxed.

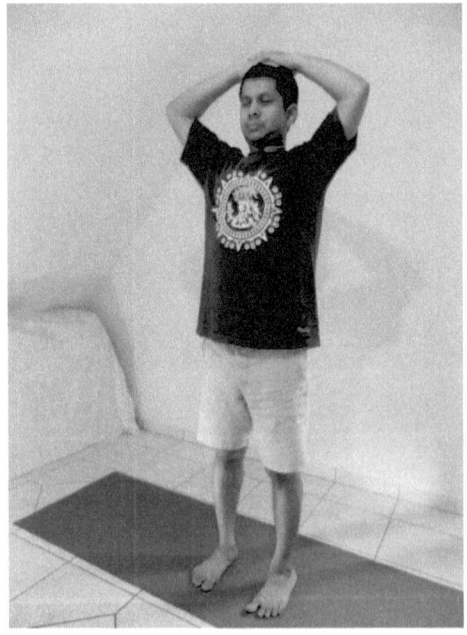

Figure 7

Drop your hands and put them by your sides. Inhale in this position. As you exhale, turn the upper body to your right side (fig.8) and inhale. Come to the centre, inhale, and as you exhale, turn to the opposite side (fig.9). Repeat these movements again. Keep the arms relaxed and passive, as if you are throwing the arms from your shoulder blades, feel how this simple movement is connected to your hips and ankles, the swing in the arms when we walk is very important for our balance. Use this swinging moves from pelvis to arms while you walk in daily life. Do this playfully 10 to 20 times without exhaustion.

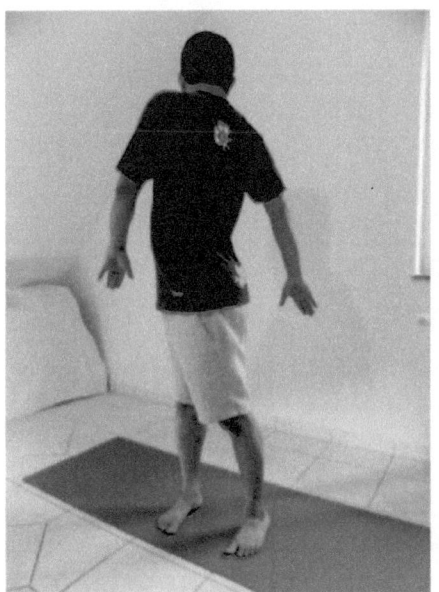 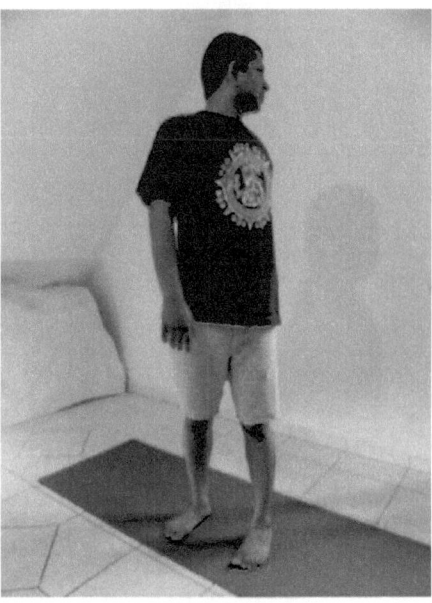

Figure 8   Figure 9

Now, we will coordinate our hands. As you exhale, turn to the left and keep your right hand on your left shoulder and your left hand on the right hip, reaching around your back (fig.10). Inhale, and then come to the centre. Stretch your hands to the side, and as you exhale, keep your left hand on your right shoulder and your right hand over the left hip (fig.11). Inhale, and then come to the centre. Continue repeating this twisting pattern. Afterwards, drop your hands to the sides of your body. Repeat this 5 to 10 times on each side. Turning the head softly, looking over the shoulder and learning to keep the spine straight and long through out the practice is important.

The twist movement is coming from the middle of the spine and proper use of ribs coordination is a key factor. Feel which shoulder blade is active and which armpit is soft.

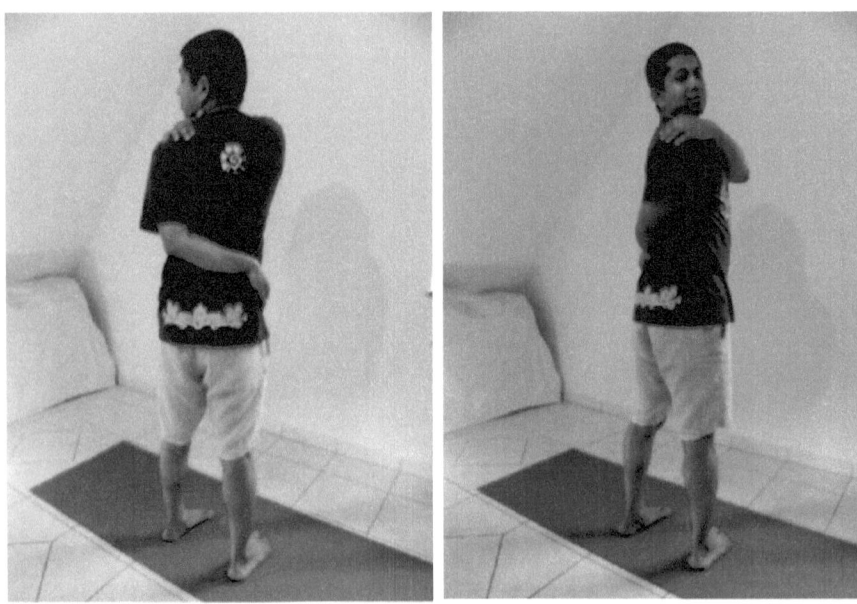

Figure 10   Figure 11

Next, turn your palms upward and pull your elbows back, closing your hands into fists in front of your chest (fig. 12). As you pull your elbows back, inhale, opening your chest. Exhale as you turn your hands so that the knuckles face upward, open the fists, and you're your hands straight forward (fig. 13). This pushes the abdomen towards your spine. Repeat these motions, making sure to inhale and exhale as you feel your abdomen move.

Abdomen muscles and organs are very important for our rhythm and movement of our legs. Repeat this movement for 10 to 15 times.

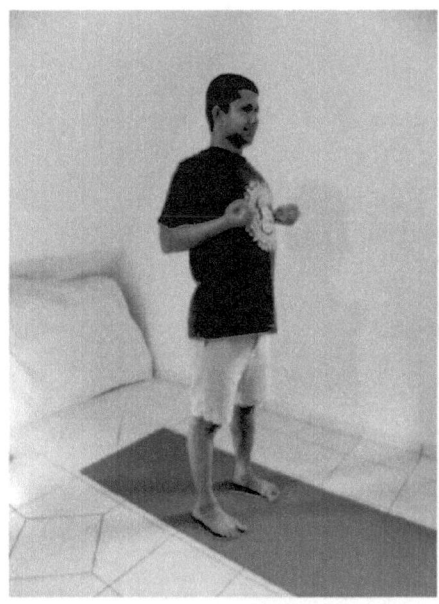 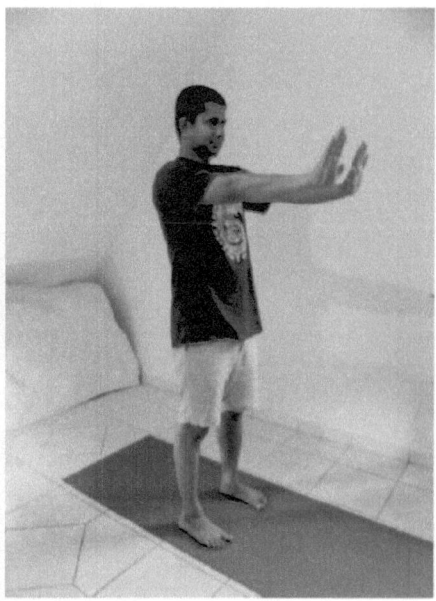

Figure 12   Figure 13

Now please open your eyes, and concentrate at a point on the ground. Spread your arms to your sides. Lift your left knee slowly so that the sole of your left food is against your right ankle. Slowly raise your left foot until it is touching the side of your right knee (fig. 14). Use your hands to balance on your right foot, and stay concentrated on the ground.

Slowly lower your arms and your left leg, and then switch legs before repeating this process.

It is very difficult to balance in one leg, even I have seen, top fit sports persons also is not good with one leg balances. Do not think whether you can balance or not, trying to communicate to brain with gravity in a different way is more important than achieving the one leg balance. Take the support of the wall if necessary, Hold the posture for 30 secconds on each leg.

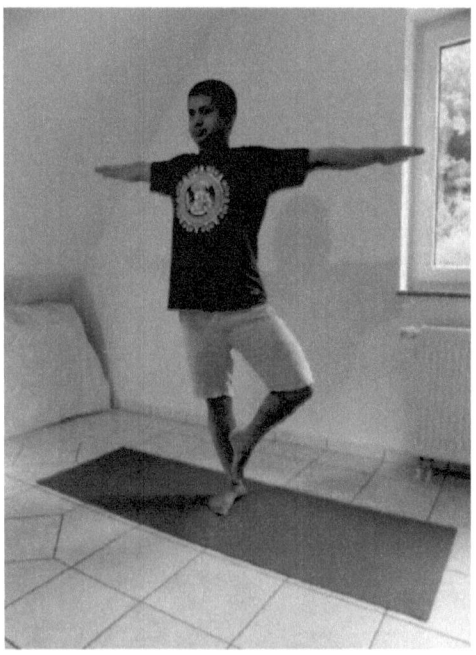

Figure 14

Improving Walking (Steps)

Stand on the mat, feeling it with the soles of your feet. Close your eyes, bend your knees, and walk backwards, feeling the mat beneath your feet (fig.15). Stop when you reach the end of the mat, and bend forward at the waist. Place your palms flat on the mat, and walk to the front of the mat with your hands and legs outstretched (fig.16). Stand up straight, close your eyes, and walk back to the end of the mat before repeating the exercise again.Yoga Sun Salutations in new format for Parkinson patients. Do this back and forth for 3 to 4 times.

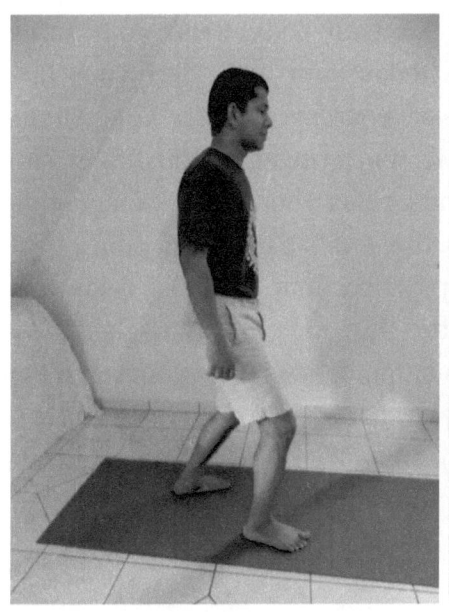 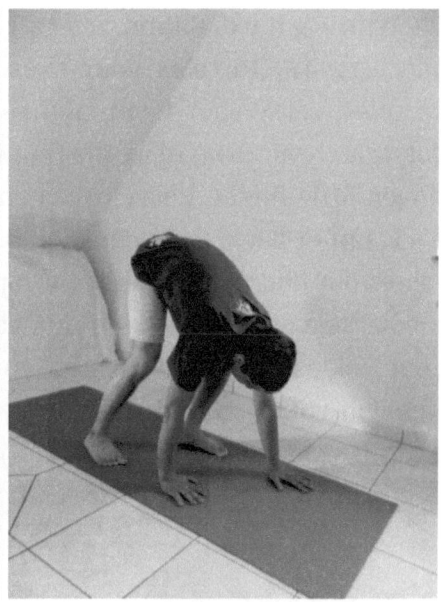

Figure 15   Figure 16

Relaxing the Muscles and the Body

Slowly lie on the mat in the dead man posture, legs apart, hands apart, and palms facing up. Close your eyes. With each exhalation, try to relax the whole body (fig.17).

Lift your right leg two inches up from the floor - stretch, stretch, and drop. Lift your left leg two inches up from the floor - stretch, stretch, and drop. Lift your right hand two inches up from the floor - stretch, stretch and drop. Repeat this process with your left hand, your hips, and your chest. Then, lift and stretch both hands and both legs.

Stretch your tongue out of your mouth. Open your eyes wide and stretch them. Look up, down, left, right. Make an ugly face by squeezing the face muscles. Make a fist. Squeeze your toes. Contract your knees. Tense all the muscles of the body, tense, tense, tense. And release.

With each exhalation, try to relax your body. Relax your hands and legs. Try to relax your eyes. Relax your lips, relax your face muscles, relax your head, and relax your neck. Relax your shoulder, relax your arm, relax the thumb, index finger, middle finger, ring finger, little finger. Relax your hands, relax your lower back, middle back, upper back, and spine. Relax the whole back, relax your chest, relax your abdomen, relax your hips, relax your buttocks, relax your thighs, relax the knees, and relax the shin and cough muscles. Relax your ankles, feet, and toes. In your mind, repeat to yourself: *I am relaxing your body. My body is relaxed. I am relaxing my mind. My mind is relaxed. I am relaxing my soul. My soul is relaxed.* Slowly begin moving again, starting with your fingers and toes.

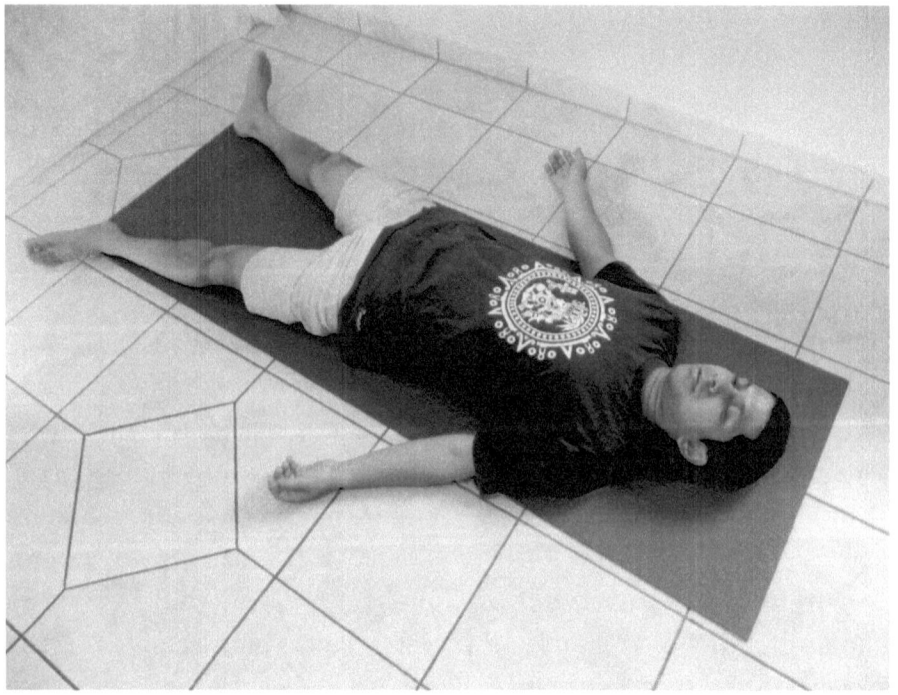

Figure 17

Massaging Your Digestive Organs

Bend your knees, keeping the soles of your feet on the mat. The right hand should be on the navel and the left hand should be on the middle of the chest. Inhale, and the abdomen comes up (fig.18) and exhale, letting the abdomen settle down towards the spine (fig.19). Repeat this process of breathing and feel your abdomen move. Now, as you inhale, pull the anus towards your naval. Relax as you exhale. Continue this pattern of breathing as you squeeze and release the anus muscles.

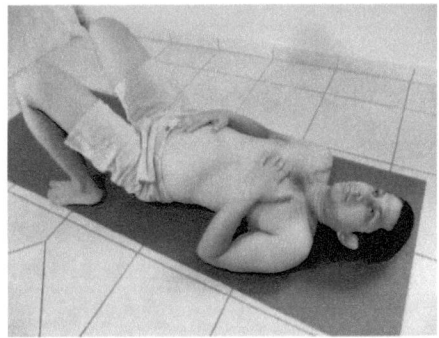 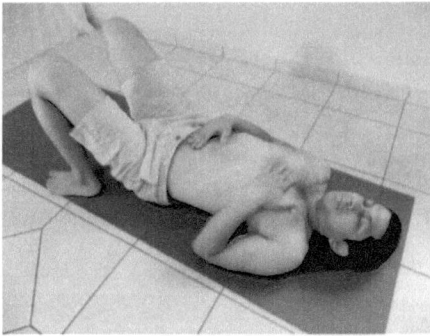

Figure 18   Figure 19

Slowly straighten your legs and join them together while lying on your back. As you exhale, bend your right knee. Pull it towards your chest and massage your digestive organs. Do the same with your left leg, and again exhale as you pull your knee towards your chest. Do this again with both legs (fig. 20) and push down slightly, massaging your digestive organs (fig.21). Inhale, and relax the legs, letting them drop down. Exhale, continuing to massage your digestive organs. Inhale, letting your legs drop.

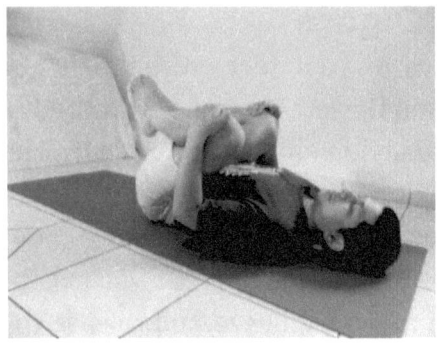 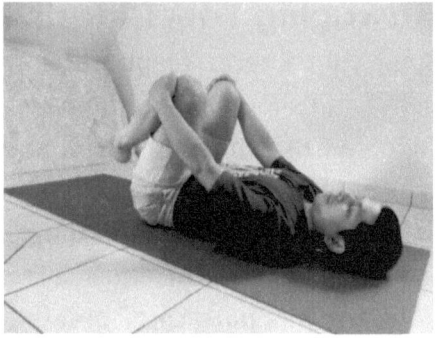

Figure 20   Figure 21

Now, place your legs together while still lying on the mat, bending them at the knee but keeping your soles on the mat. Press your inner thighs together as you stretch your hands to your side, level with your shoulders. As you exhale, drop both knees to your left, and turn your head to the right. Inhale as you come to the center, As you exhale, drop your knees to your right side, turning your head to the left. Repeat this exercise (fig.22) several times, alternating sides.

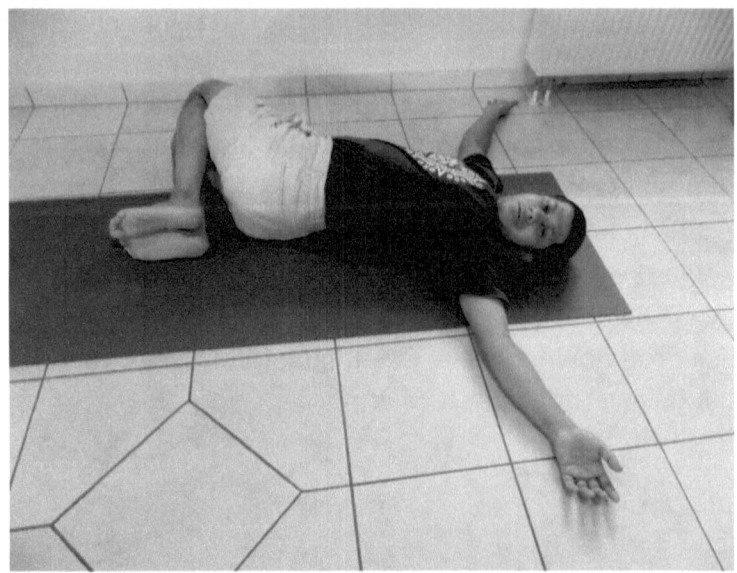

Figure 22

Placing your hands on your knees, you can rotate your lower back and massge your digestion organs(fig 23).

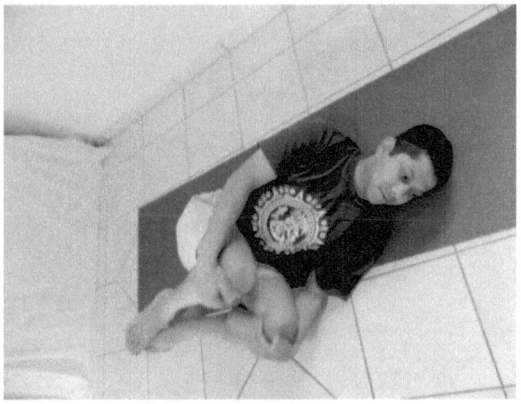

Figure 23

How to Improve Rolling and Body Reflexes

While lying on your back, pull your knees to your chest, leaving your hands on your knees. Inhale while at the center (fig.24) As you exhale, drop the whole body to the left side(fig25). Again inhale, come into the centre and as you exhale, drop the whole body to the right side. Repeat this a few more times, alternating sides.

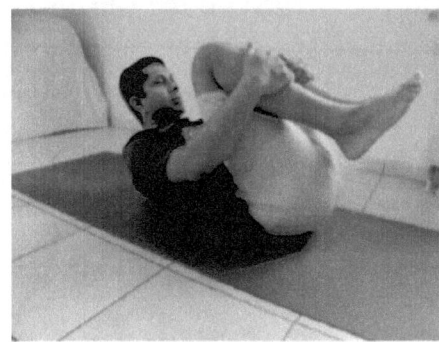 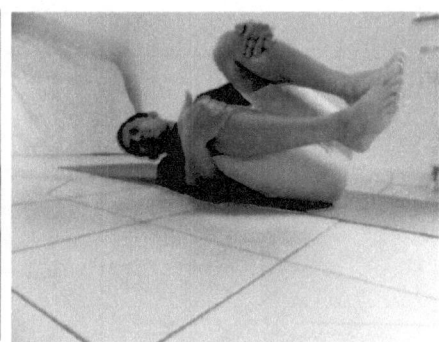

Figure 24   Figure 25

This movement will help you to turn in the bed in a better way, use this movement to turn in the bed easily. Again come into centre, now with your neck and back elevated. Rock back and forth like a rocking chair (fig.26,fig.27) After you do this several times, come out and relax in the dead man's posture - separate the legs apart - palms facing up. With each exhalation, relax the whole body and release the weight of your body to the floor.

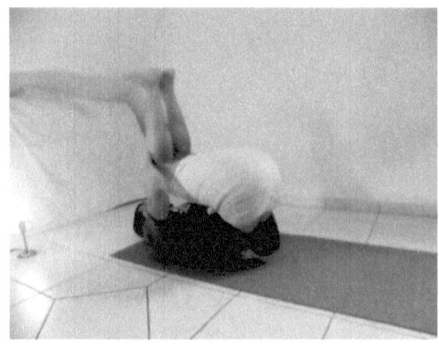
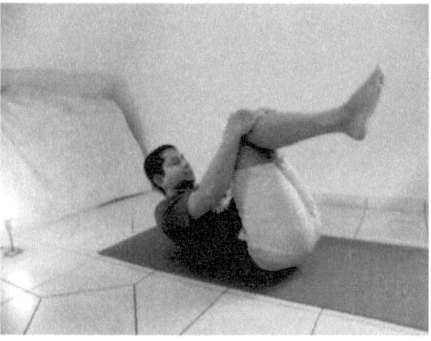

Figure 26   Figure 27

Flexible Back

Slowly turn your body so that you're lying on your abdomen, elbows on the mat and palms just under your chin. Join your legs together. As you exhale, bend the right leg from the knee (fig.28) Inhale, dropping the leg down and allowing it to relax. Then do the same with your left leg(fig.29) Don't forget to exhale as you bend the leg and inhale as you drop it down.

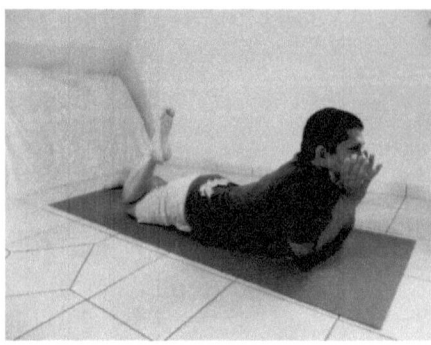
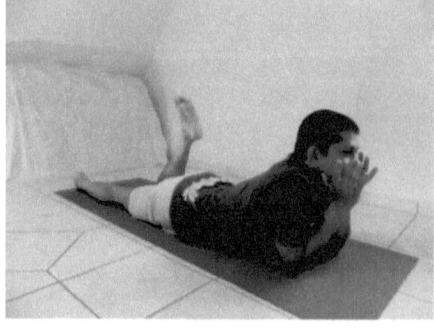

Figure 28   Figure 29

Place your palms on the mat underneath your shoulders, elbows pointing up. Join your legs together and place your chin on the mat. Lift your chin up, opening up your chest. Look up, and exhale. Place your chin on the mat, and again inhale as you come up into the cobra position. Exhale as you move your chest back down, and repeat this exercise (fig.30, fig31,fig32,fig 33).

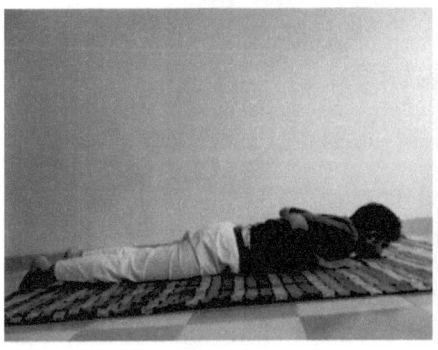
Figure 30

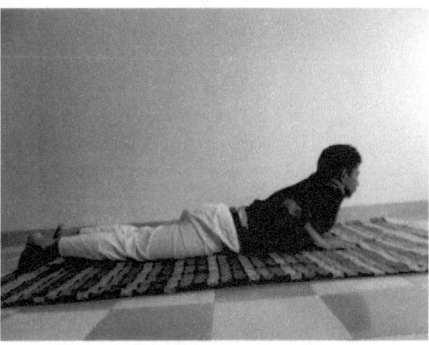
Figure 31

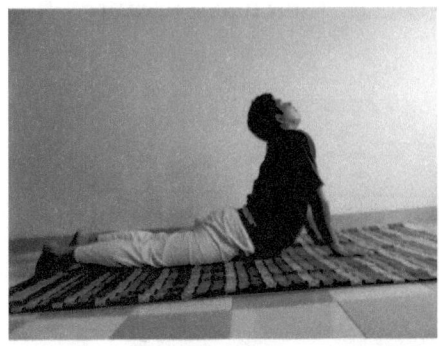
Figure 32

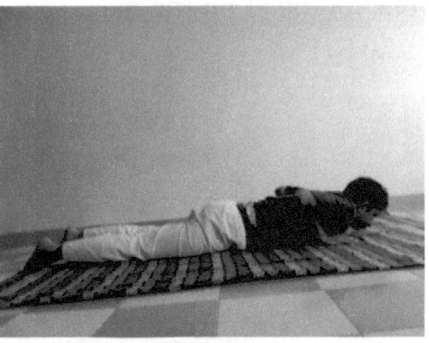
Figure 33

Now, slowly come down, and place one hand on top of the other under your head, making a pillow for your forehead. Relax your legs, spreading them a little. As you inhale, push your abdomen onto the mat. Exhale, relaxing the abdomen. Repeat this breathing pattern, making sure to feel your abdomen's movements (fig34).

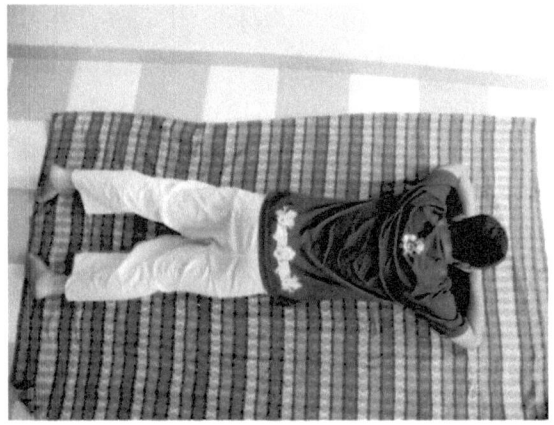

Figure 34

Now, slowly come out of this pose and place your palms on the mat under your shoulders, your big toes touching each other with your heels apart. Push your body back so that your buttocks rest on your heels. Your hands should be to your sides, by your ankles, with your forehead on the mat. This is called "the child's posture." (Fig. 35,36,37)

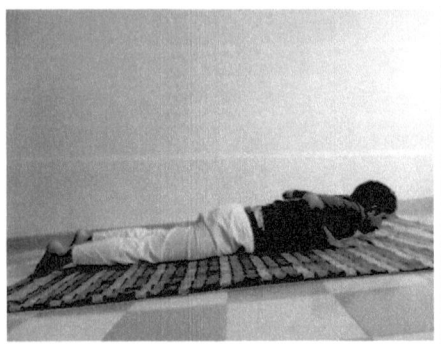

Figure 35

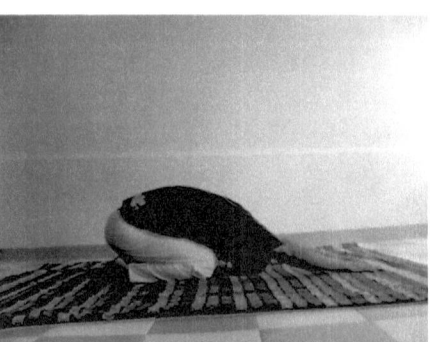

Figure 36

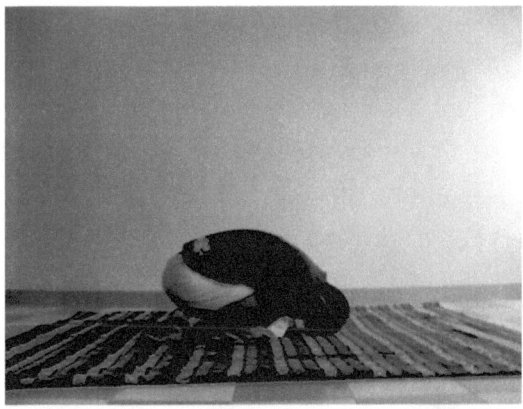

Figure 37

Relax in this pose for a while, and when you're ready, lift your chest out and stand on your knees. Walk with your knees until you are in the middle of your mat. Separate the knees a little so that you can balance on them. Keep your hands on your lower back, and as you exhale, drop your head back so that the abdomen is pushed to the front. Exhale, and come into a normal standing position. Again, inhale and lean back. Drop your head down and exhale, coming into an upright position. For the last time, drop the head back, and again push the abdomen out towards your front. (Fig. 38, Fig.39)

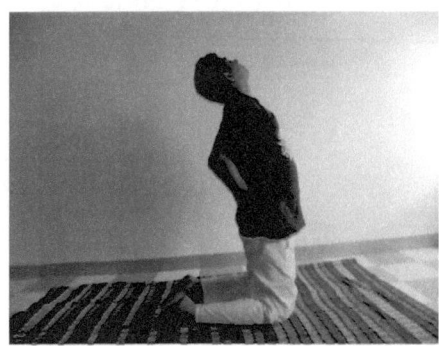 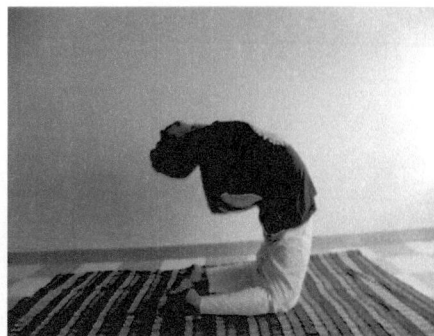

Figure 38   Figure 39

Now, drop your hands onto the mat so that your arms form a 90 degree angle. As you inhale, drop your abdomen towards the mat.

and lift your head up. Look up, just like a cow, and when you exhale, lift the middle of your back up toward the sky and put your head towards the mat, just like a cat. Inhale into the cow pose, and exhale into the cat pose. As you continue alternating between these positions, feel the movement of your spine as it comes into alignment with your head. (Fig 40, Fig.41)

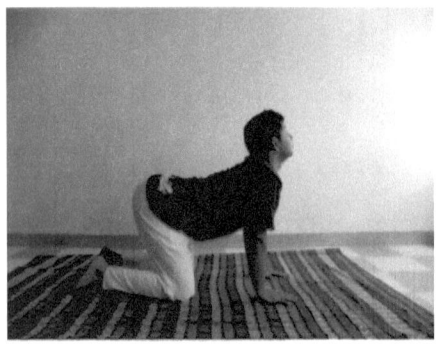

Figure 40

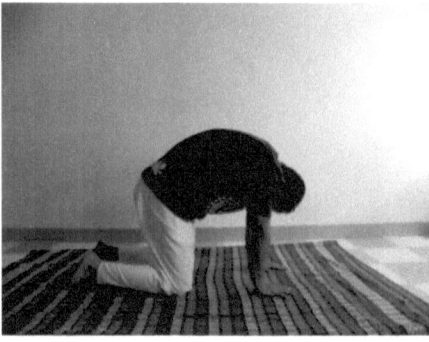

Figure 41

Next, inhale and stretch your right leg back so that it's directly behind you. As you exhale, drop the knee back onto the mat. Now, inhale as you lift your left leg and stretch it back. Exhale as you slowly move your knee back to the mat. Repeat this movement several times, alternating legs.(Fig.42)

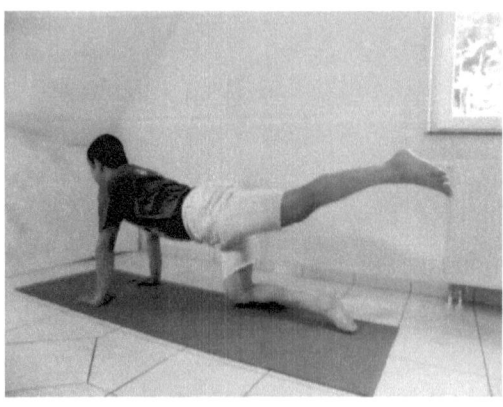

Figure 42

Now, inhale and stretch your right arm forward and your left leg backward. Exhale as you return your knee and hand to the mat. Repeat this as you inhale again, this time lifting your left arm and right leg. After you stretch them out, exhale as your arm and leg return to the mat. (Fig43) Repeat this 5 to 10 times on each side, good for balance & coordinating the arms and legs also.

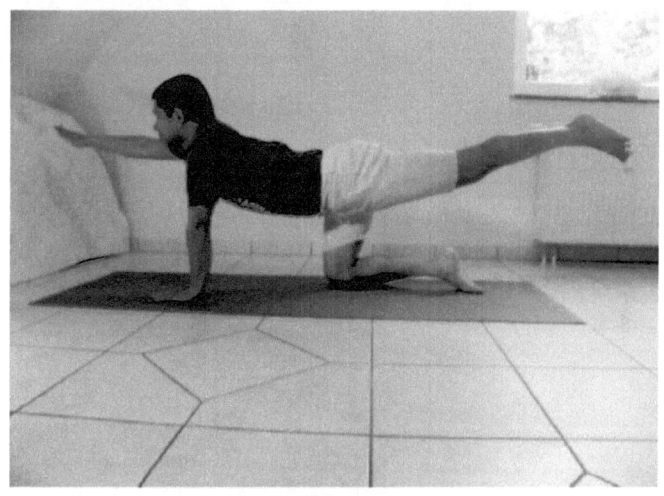

Figure 43

Place your buttocks on your heels again. Stretch your hands out in front of you, place your forehead on the mat, and allow your body to relax. (Fig.36)

Improving Motor Function and Range of Motion

Slowly sit up and then stretch your legs in front of you(Fig44). Place your hands behind you for support. Put your legs together, and as you exhale, squeeze the muscles in your toes (fig.45) Relax your toes as you inhale. (fig.46)

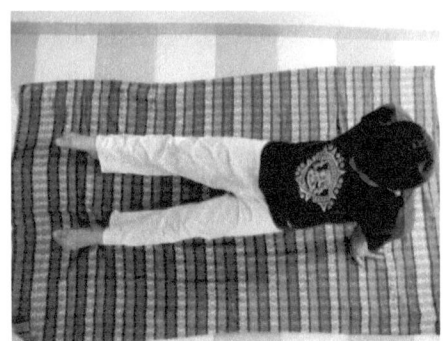
Figure 44

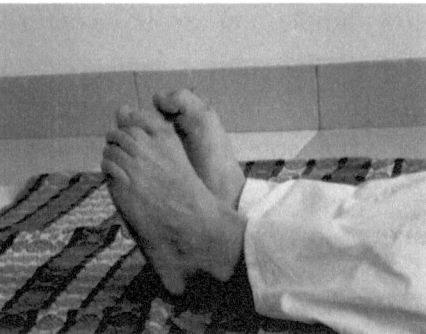
Figure 45

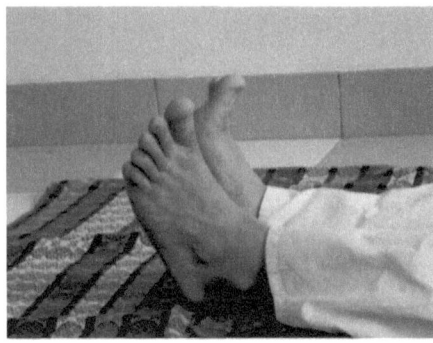
Figure 46

Stretch the ankles and inhale, toes pointing towards the body. Exhale, stretch the ankles and inhale, toes pointing towards the body... (fig.47,fig.48)

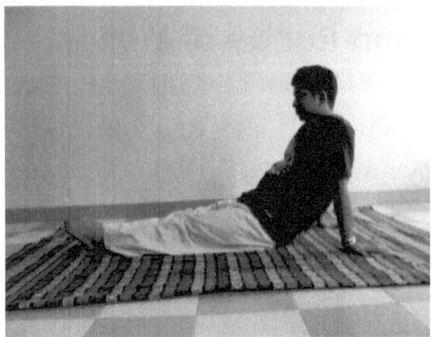
Figure 47

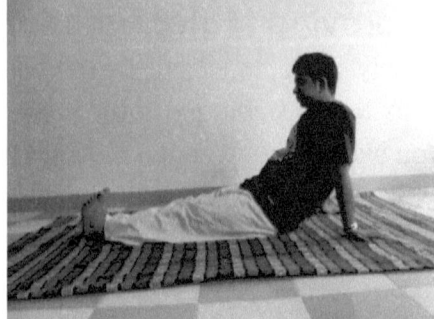
Figure 48

Now rotate your ankles, breathe comfortably, and then rotate your ankles in the opposite direction.

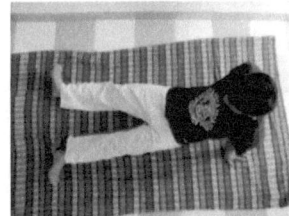 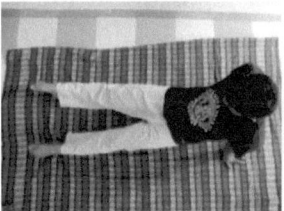 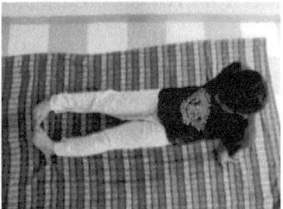

Figure 49 a,b,c

Next, bend the right leg, grab the thighs by interlocking your fingers under the thigh, and rotate the knee joint. Make a big circle with your right leg, and then rotate it in the opposite direction.(fig.50 a,b,c) Relax the right leg, and then do the same with your left leg, making sure to rotate in each direction..

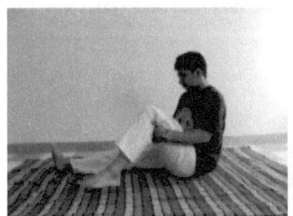 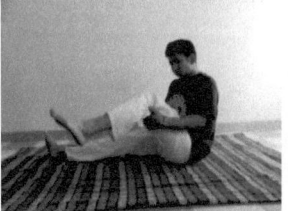 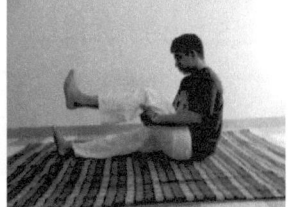

Figure 50 a,b,c

After this, grab the thigh by interlocking your fingers under the thighs, and rotate the hip in each direction. Do the same with your right hip joint and then the left before returning to center. (Fig 51 a,b,c)

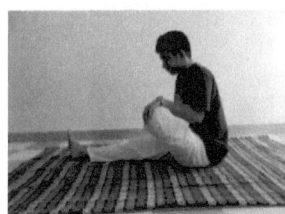 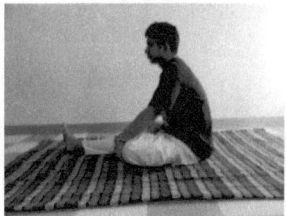 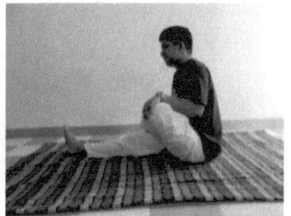

Figure 51 a,b,c

Join the soles of your feet together and flap your knees up and down like the wings of a butterfly. Open up your hip joints through movement before relaxing your legs and sitting in a comfortable posture, using a pillow or chair if necessary. (Fig 52 a,b,c)

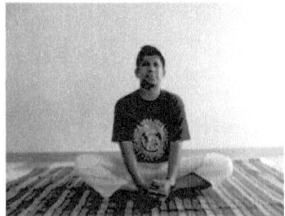 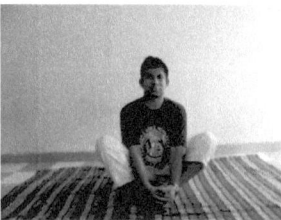 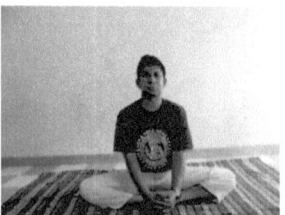

Figure 52 a,b,c

Stretch your hands to your sides as you inhale. Exhale as you relax your hands and shoulders. Repeat these movements, feeling your chest stretch and open as you inhale(fig53). And exhale relax the stretch,open the chest and ribs by extending the shoulder joints repeat 5 to 10 times.

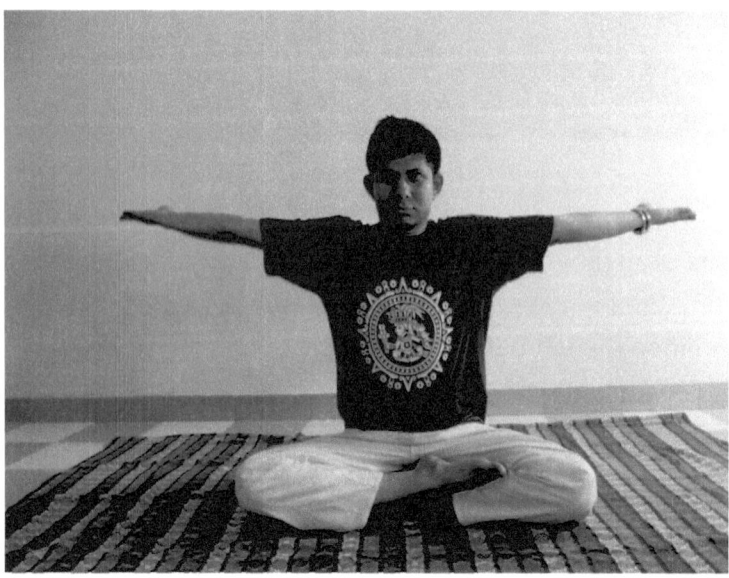

Figure 53

Place you fingers on your shoulder joints, rotating them in each direction(fig.54 a,b,c) open the ribs and give space to lungs and heart. Please repeat 5 to 10 times in one direction then change the direction, rotate in the opposite direction.

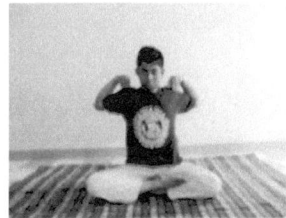 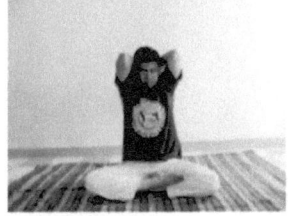 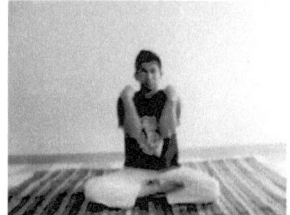

Figure 54 a,b,c

Next, slowly rotate your head,(fig.55 a,b,c) relaxing your neck, and then switch directions.

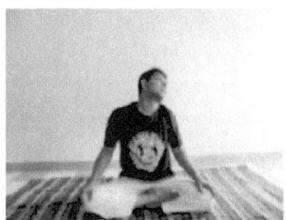 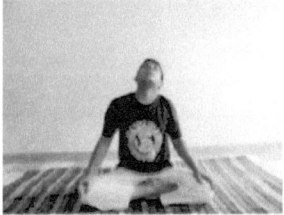 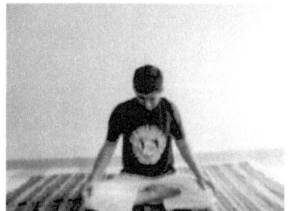

Figure 55 a,b,c

Raise your head back to center and, keeping your head still, rotate your eyeballs in each direction. Slowly close your eyes, and rub your palms together, generating heat. Cup your eyeballs, soaking up their energy. Rub the palms on your face, neck, throat, chest, abdomen, thighs, and then slowly open your eyes. Eye movements have direct relation with neck, ribs and your legs,if one feels this connection movements, turning and balance become easier.

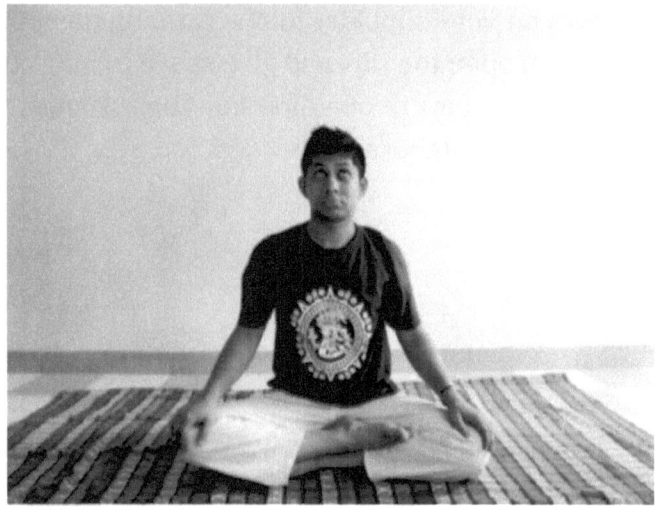

Figure 56

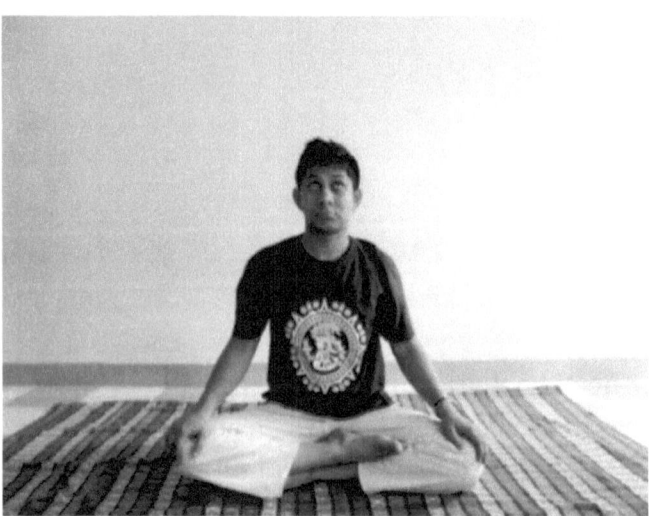

Figure 57

Now as you inhale join your hands together and as you exhale join the tips of the finger together. When you inhale, join the tips of your finger together. Repeat this for 5 to 10 times.(fig.58 a,b)

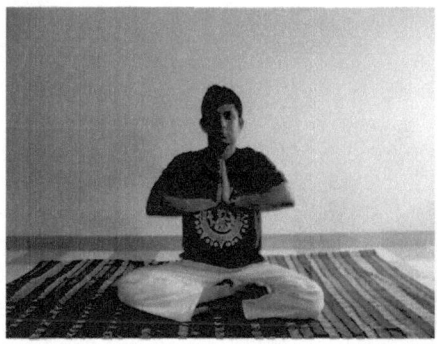 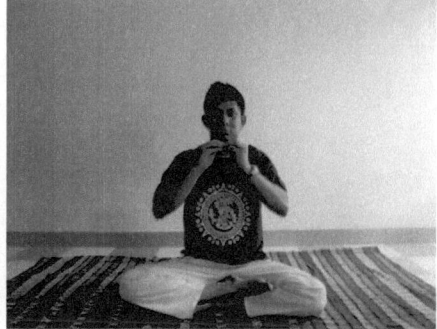

Figure 58 a,b

Improving your Facial Expression, Swallowing, and Drooling (Face Yoga)

Push your lips out as though you are kissing the air, like a pig's face. Do five times(fig.59)

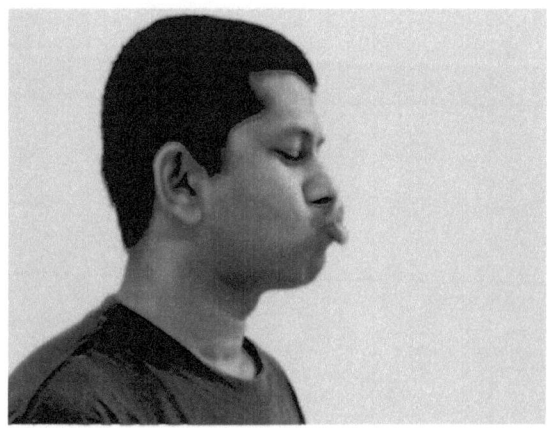

Figure 59

Turn the lips inside, close it and put air in your cheeks, make a face like a monkey. Repeat 5 times. (Fig.60)

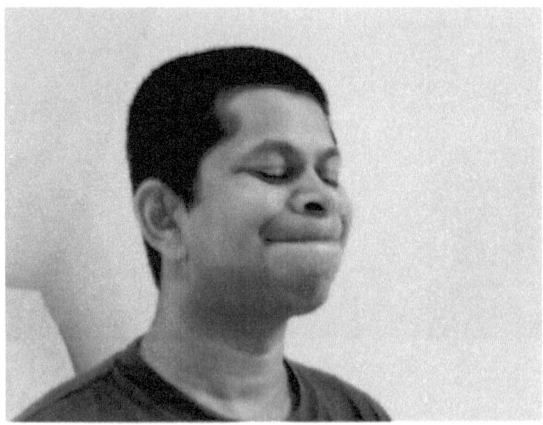

Figure 60

Now make the face like a chimpanzee by turning down your lower lip.Do 5 times (fig.61)

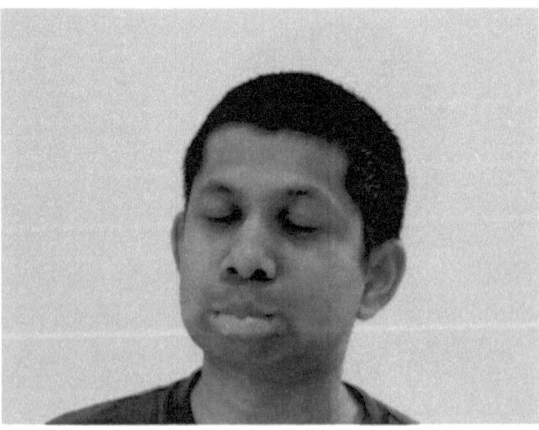

Figure 61

Next, make a face like a rabbit by pushing your upper teeth out, and act as though you're eating a carrot. Have Fun and practice for 30 seconds.(fig.62)

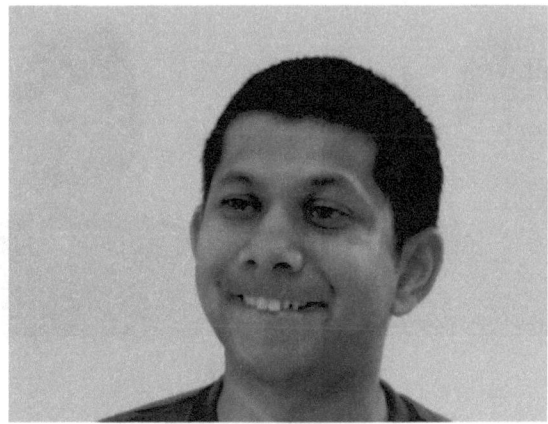

Figure 62

Let your tongue loll out of your mouth like a dog, breathing deeply. Practice for 30 seconds.(fig.63)

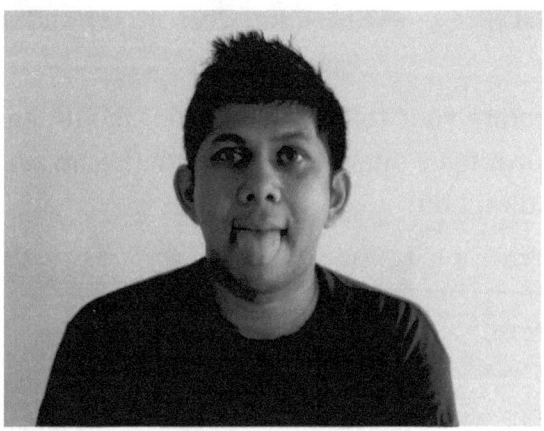

Figure 63

Make strange faces, and allow yourself to play with your eyes, lips, cheeks, nose, tongue, and ears. Allow your body to make

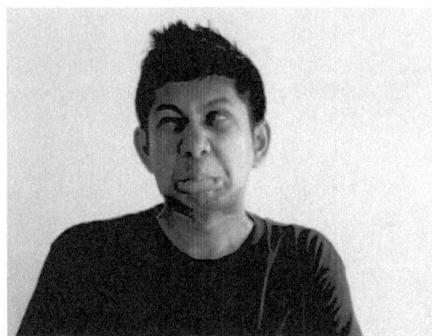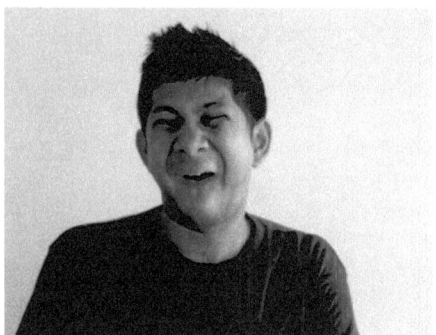

Figure 64 a,b

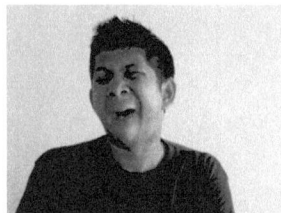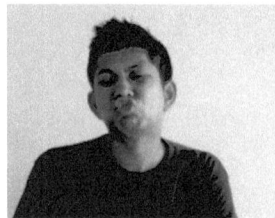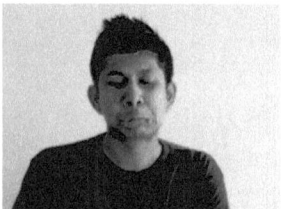

Figure 65 a,b,c

noises. Now rotate your tongue inside your mouth and then do the same with your tongue outside your mouth.(Fig.66 a,b,c, d,e) 5 to 10 times in each direction.

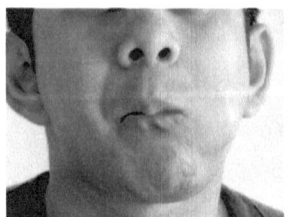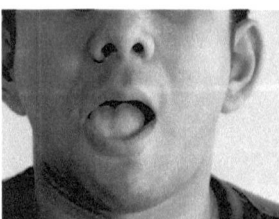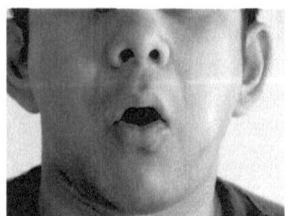

Figure 66 a,b,c

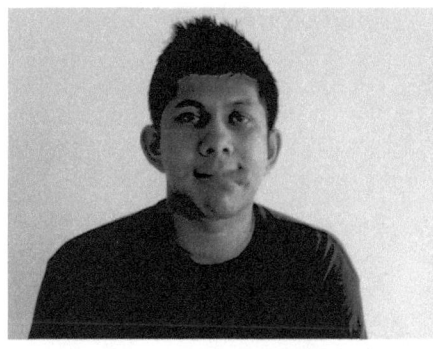 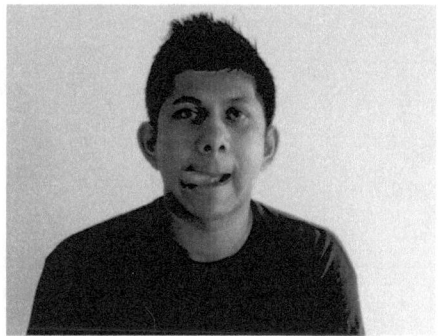

Figure 66 d,e

Vibrate your lips, creating a motorcycle-like sound.(Fig.67)

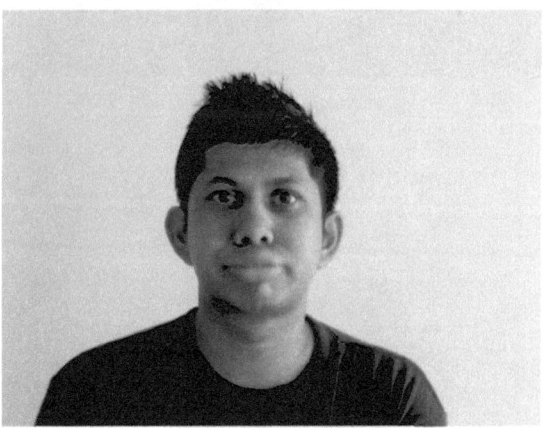

Figure 67

Relax your facial muscles, and then feel the air with your mouth. Clap your cheeks with your palms(fig.68)

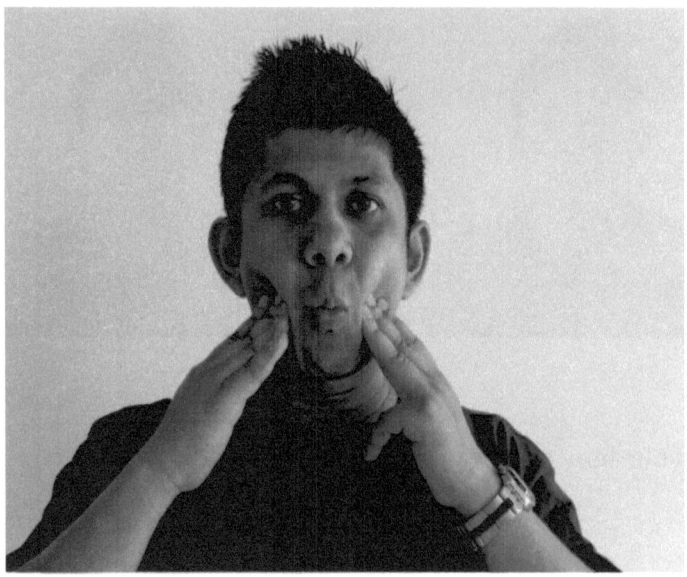

Figure 68

Next, whistle. The sound it makes is less important than the facial movements.

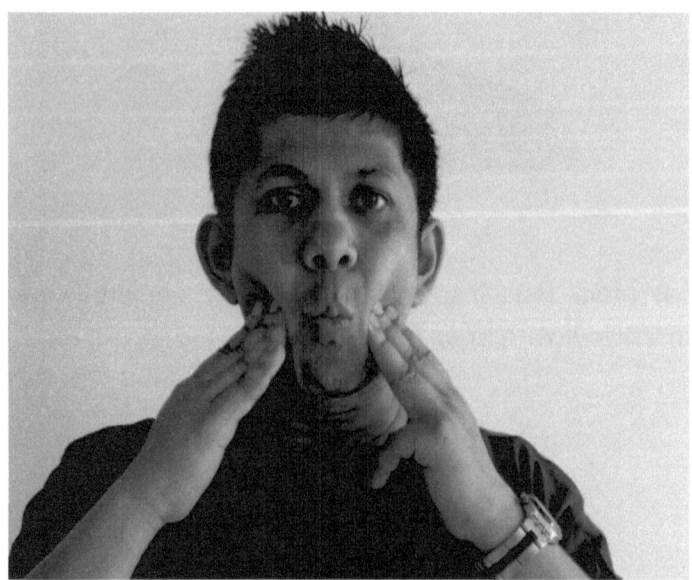

Figure 69

Reducing Depression and Improving Voice Quality (Laughter Yoga)

Laughing too much is not good for parkinson patients,from my experience I have noticed that too much laughter is not good for the nervous system for the Parkinson patients.If one has heart problem or Mental disorder be careful.

Its increases vata according to Ayurveda. Do this laughing exercises only for 30 sec to 1 minute maximum. Just use this laughing exercises to understand the connection of upper body muscles, organs and diaphragm that produces the wind play and voice quality, as and actor or singer improvises the vocal tone, but in a funny way. Laugh with your abdomen, and place your hand over your abdomen so that you can feel the movement as you do so. *Ha ha ha.*

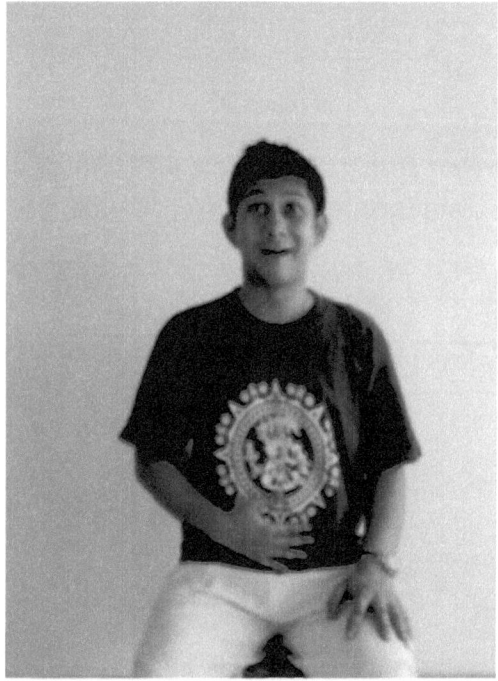

Figure 70 a

Laugh with your chest, and feel the movement of your lungs. *Ha ha ha.*

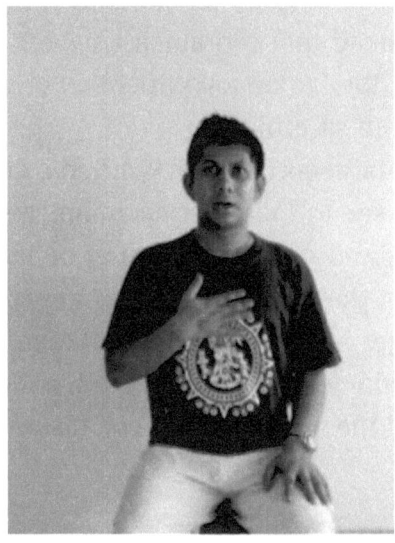

Figure 70 b

Now laugh with your throat, Use your vocal chords and try to create many kinds of sound through your throat. *Ho ho ho.*

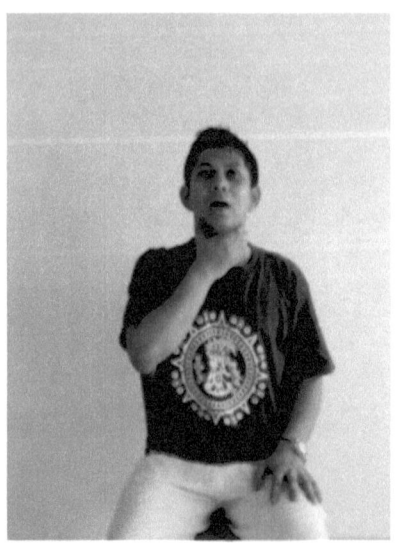

Figure 70 c

Laugh with your mouth, use the facial muscles, the inner mouth space to create the laughter.

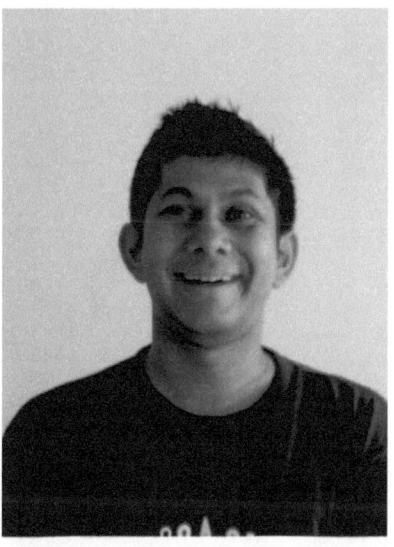

Figure 70 d

Then laugh with your nose, just like a horse as if you are blowing your nose.

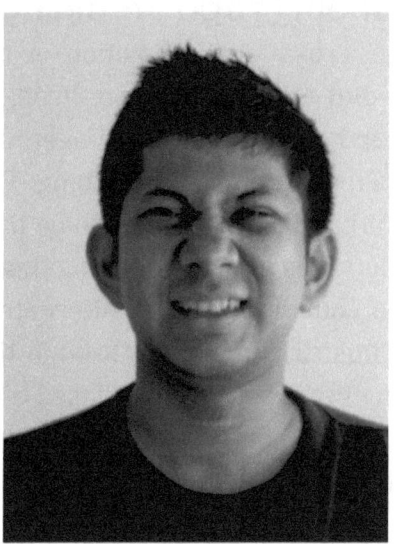

Figure 70 e

Open your eyes, and laugh spontaneously, naturally. *Ha ha ho ho hee hee hee.* Spread your legs and hands, and allow laughter to consume your entire body. Then relax for a while, let the breath calm down.

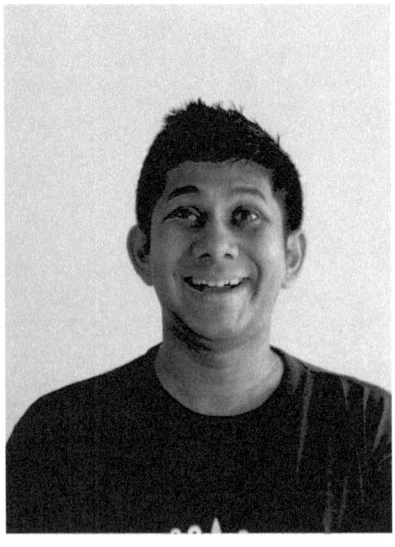

Figure 70 f

Stress Management (Yoga Breathing)

Sit in a comfortable, cross-legged position or any other comfortable sitting posture.But keep your spine, head, and neck Straight. Using your Right hand thumb and ring finger, close one nostril at a time to practice alternate nostril breathing. First close the right nostril with the right hand's thumb and inhale through the left nostril. Then close the left nostril with your ring finger, as you open the right exhale through your right nostril. Alternate so that you inhale through your right nostril and exhale through the left. Repeat this three times, ensuring that your lips are closed and that your inhalations are deep and long. To perfect this ask a yoga teacher to show you the proper method.

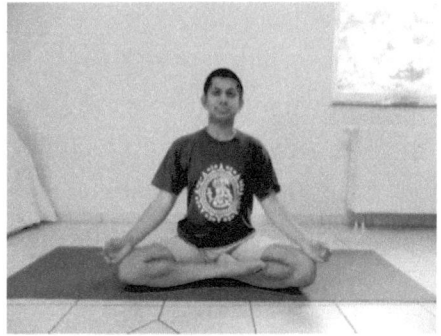

Figure 71

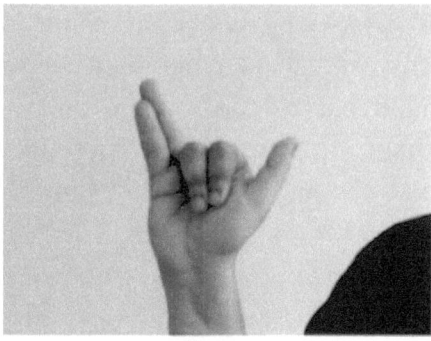

Figure 72

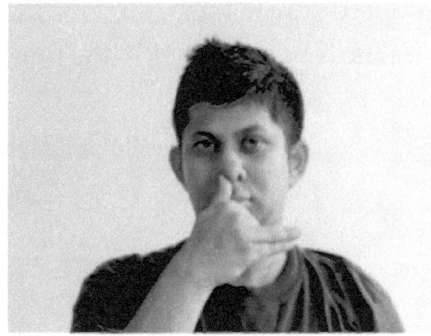

Figure 73

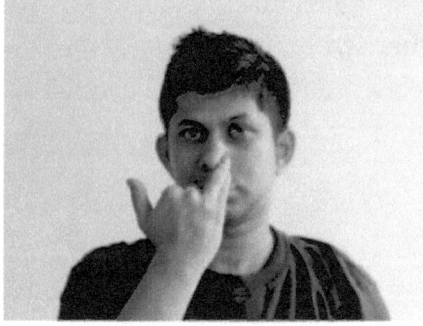

Figure 74

Inhale through the nose and then plug your ears with your index fingers. As you exhale, keep your lips closed and hum like a humming bee. Repeat this two or three times before slowly dropping your hands back to your sides.

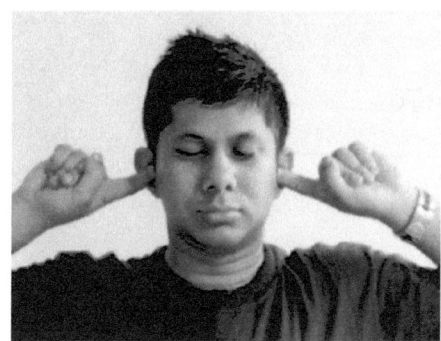

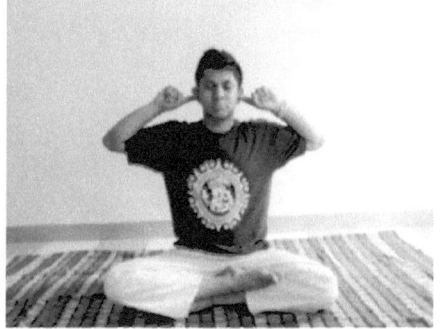

Figure 75 a,b

Improving Cognitive Function (Meditation)

Now we will do a meditation using finger coordination to relax your mind and feel the peace within. We will coordinate our fingers as we chant: A, U, M, E. Join the thumb and the index finger and say "A," then the middle finger and say "U," and the ring finger and say "M," and on the small finger, say "E." Keep your eyes closed and your hands on your thighs with your palms facing up. A-U-M-E. A-U-M-E. Keep your eyes closed and feel the peace within. Smile with your eyes, lips, and cheeks until your whole face is smiling. Smile with your whole body, and as you focus on your happiness, allow your mind and soul to smile as well. Aim to stay in this state for anywhere from five to twenty minutes. If it is difficult to seat in the floor take a chair but keep the spine straight as possible.

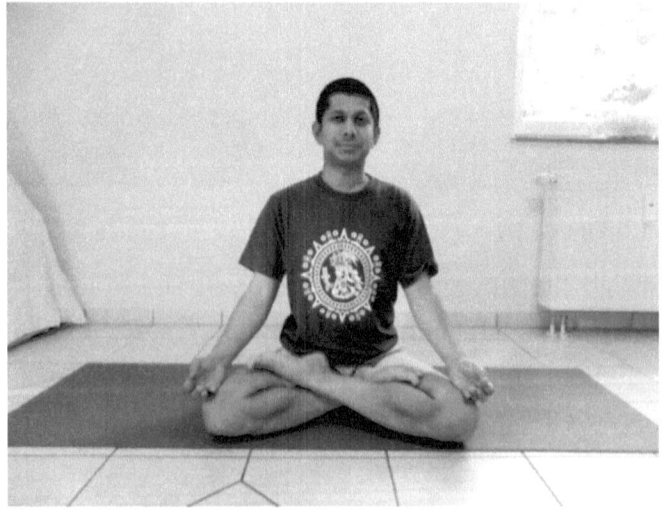

Figure 76

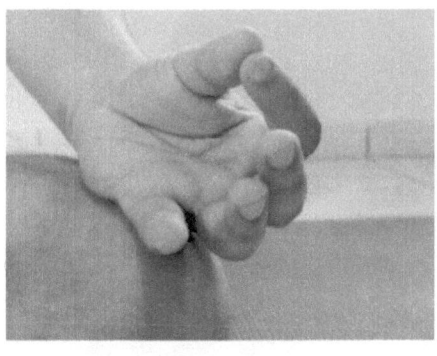
Figure 77

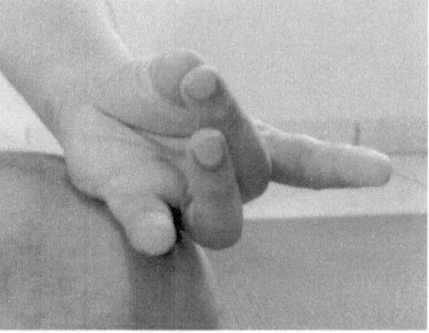
Figure 78

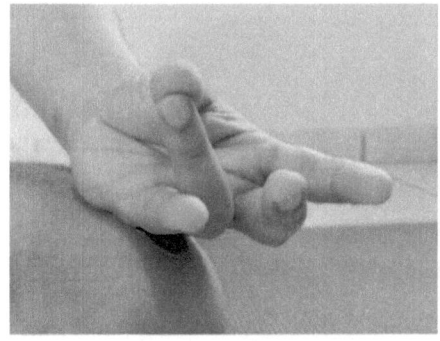
Figure 79

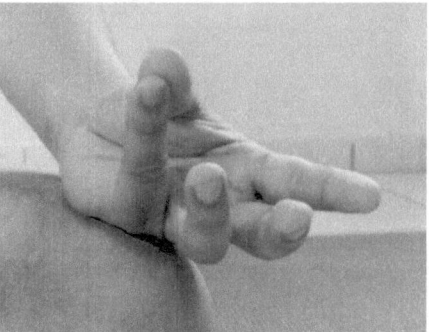
Figure 80

Yoga II

For patients who require mobility (walking stick to wheelchair) or equipment aids, or assistance in their daily activities (ATL).

Improving Motor Function & Range of Motion

Sit comfortably in a chair by keeping your spine, neck, and head straight, your chest open, and your head high. Keep the soles of your feet on the ground and place your hands on your thighs. Press both the heels on the ground and lift the toes up, giving you better control over your toes.

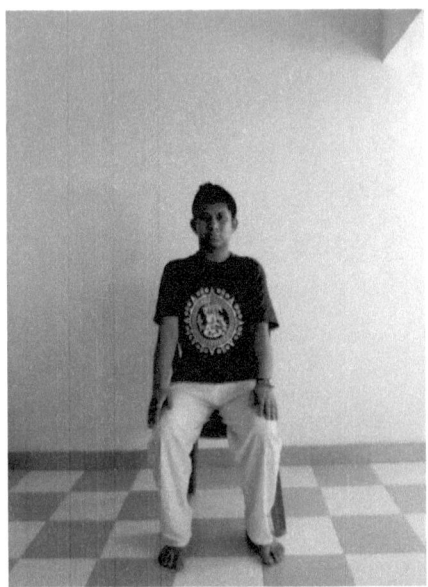 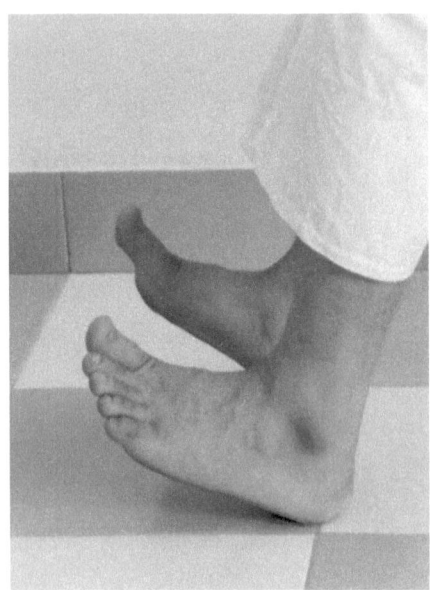

Figure 81   Figure 82

As you exhale, squeeze or turn your toes towards the floor, and as you inhale, relax the toes. Repeat this pattern of squeezing and relaxing the muscles ten times, inhaling and exhaling each time.

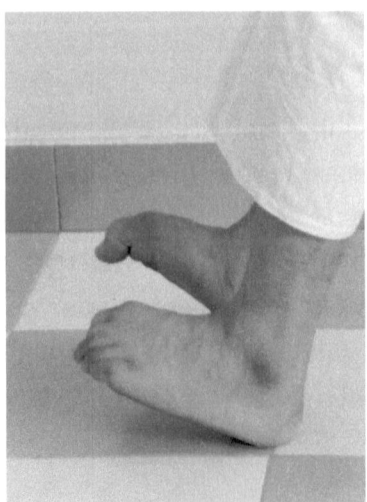

Abb. 83

Feel the bodily movements and try to find out when in your daily life you might use this movement. Throughout the day, use or imagine using these movements, and try to connect to your body and talk to it silently, like a meditation. Slowly drop the soles of your feet to the ground. Now grab your right thigh by interlocking the fingers underneath the thigh. Lift the leg a little so that your heel is 10 cm above the floor. As you exhale, stretch the right ankle, and as you inhale, turn the toes on your right foot towards the body. Exhale, stretching your feet. Inhale, turning your toes towards your body. Do this ten times.

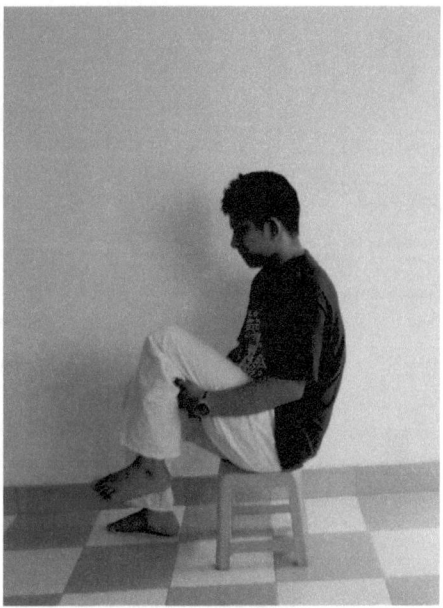

Figure 84

While sitting in the same position, rotate your right ankle. If you can't physically do this, just imagine moving your ankle without stress or pressure on the ankle joint. Rotate the ankle in the opposite direction. Repeat this exercise with your left side, beginning by squeezing the toes on your left foot as you inhale and relaxing the toes as you exhale ten times.

Grab the right leg beneath the thigh again, and rotate the right hip joint ten times in each direction, clockwise and then anticlockwise. Do the same thing with the left leg before slowly dropping it down to center.

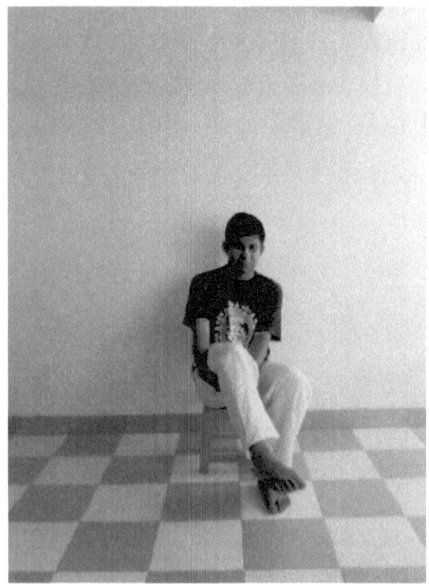

Figure 85

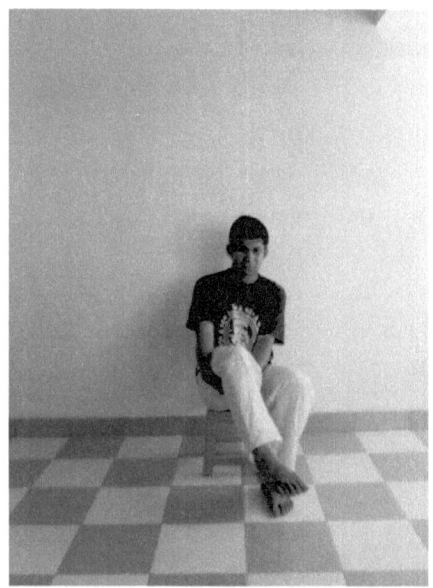

Figure 86

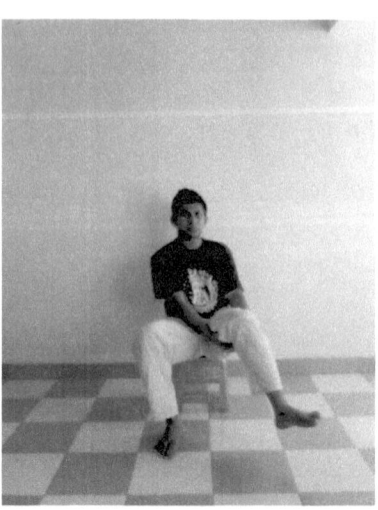

Figure 87

Flexiblity & Balance.

Sit on the front of your chair so that you have lots of space behind you to work out your spine. Keep your soles on the floor, and straighten your spine, neck, and head. Open your chest and hold your head high, placing your palms flat on your thighs.

As you inhale, push your chest out so that your shoulders are back and you're looking up, a position like a cow. As you exhale, pull the middle of your spine towards the chair, and by pressing your palms on your thighs, pull your abdomen towards your spine like a cat, bowing your head downwards in front of you. Alternate between the cow and cat positions, inhaling and exhaling each time. Do this ten times, making your spine more flexible.

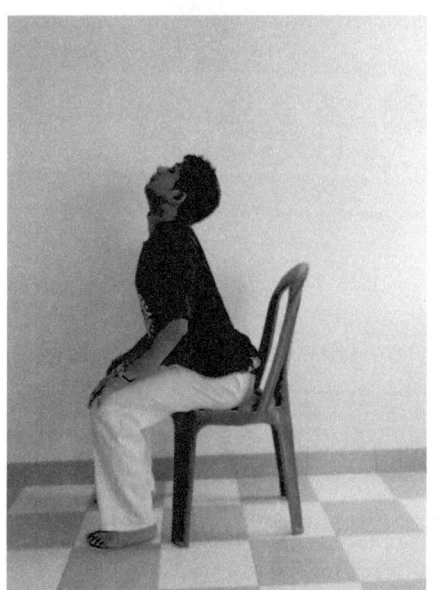
Figure 88

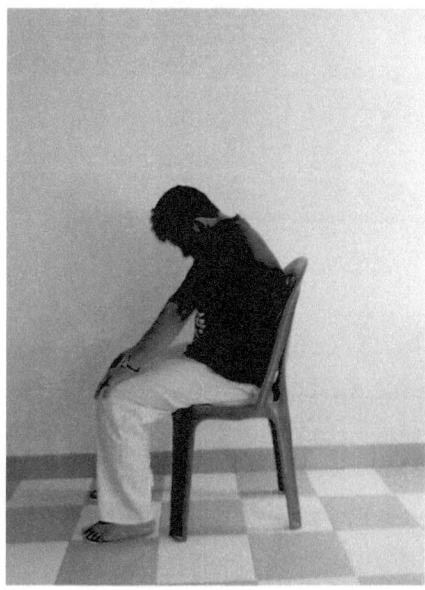
Figure 89

Sit tall by keeping your spine, neck, and head straight and the soles of your feet on the floor. You can gain better control over the upper body by pressing the soles of your feet onto the ground. Now interlock your fingers behind your head, inhale in your chest, and twist to your right side at the waist as you exhale. Inhale as you return back to the center, and exhale as you turn, this time to your left side. Repeat this exercise five times, breathing in and out as you alternate sides.

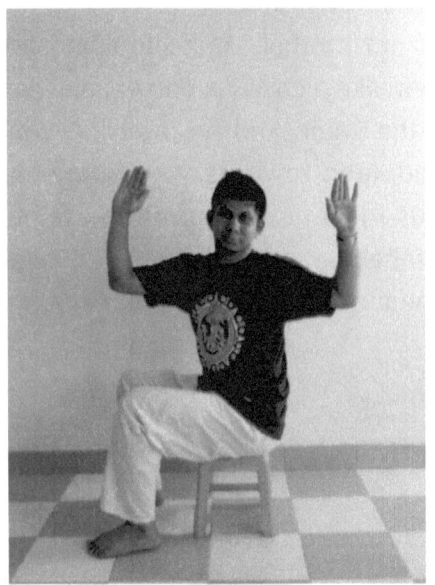 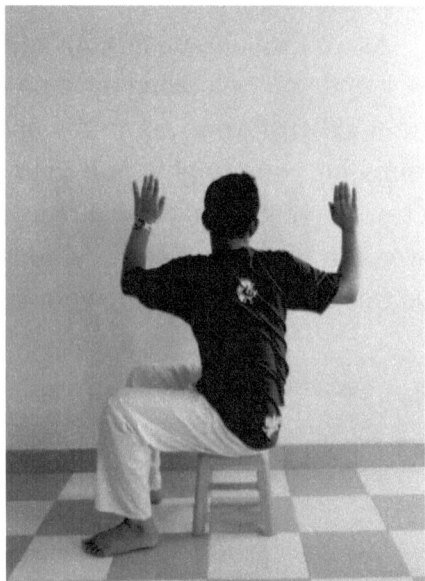

Figure 90   Figure 91

Slowly come back to center and drop your hands to your thighs. Now we will rotate the upper body by using the lower back. Rotate your head and upper body to the side, return to center, and then rotate your upper body to the other side. Keep the soles of your feet planted on the ground for better control over your upper body. Continue to rotate your body ten times in each direction.

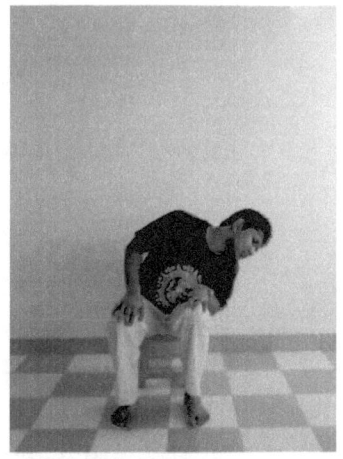

Figure 92

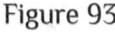

Figure 93

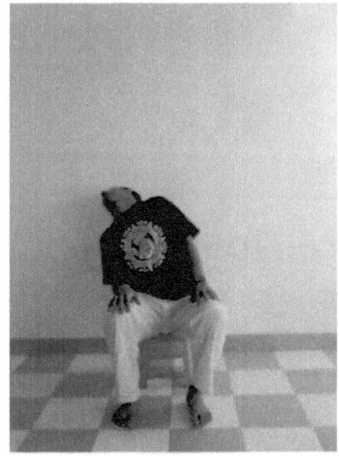

Figure 94

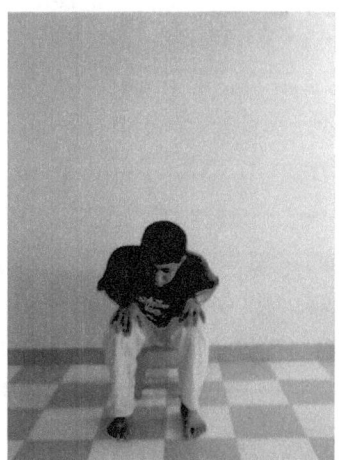

Figure 95

Relaxation

Lie back on the chair, relaxing the whole body and keeping it loose. Close your eyes; we'll now try a relaxing meditation in which we talk to each body part mentally.

With each exhalation, try to release the weight of the body to the chair, shifting your awareness. With each exhalation, relax your hands. -Inhale and focus. With your next exhalation, relax your legs.

Make them easy and loose. Try to relax your thumbs, relax the index fingers, and the middle fingers. Relax the little finger, and feel your whole hand relax.

Relax the muscles in your wrist, your lower arms, and feel the looseness spread up your arms, over the elbow. Relax your shoulders, followed by your neck, throat, and head. Think about the stress draining from your eyes, your lips, and each of your face muscles.

Allow the chest and abdomen to relax. As your belly loosens, relax your lower back, and feel the sensation spread up your back until it is entirely loose as well. Let the tension drain from your spine, hips, buttocks, thighs, and knees. Think about your whole body being relaxed from head to toe.

Mentally repeat: *I am relaxing my body. My body is relaxed. I am relaxing my mind. My mind is relaxed. I am relaxing my soul. My soul is relaxed. I am relaxed.*

Slowly begin moving the muscles in your body once you're ready, beginning with your fingers and toes.

Improving Fine Motor Function (Dexterity)

Sit at the edge of your chair with your spine, neck, and head straight, your chest open, and your chin lifted high.

Begin by rotating your shoulder joints, placing your fingers on the shoulder. If your shoulders are stiff, stretch your arms out to the side and rotate your arms. Do this ten times clockwise and ten times counterclockwise.

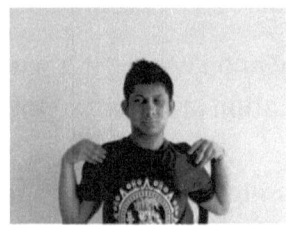 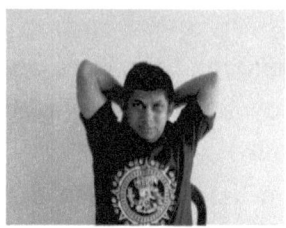 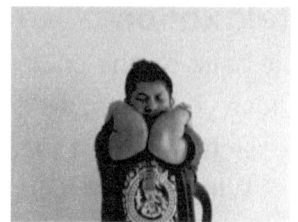

Figure 96 a,b,c

Return to the center, and rotate your head and neck slowly. If your neck is too stiff to do this comfortably, just imagine that you are doing so, picturing these movements in your mind. Rotate ten times clockwise and ten times counterclockwise.

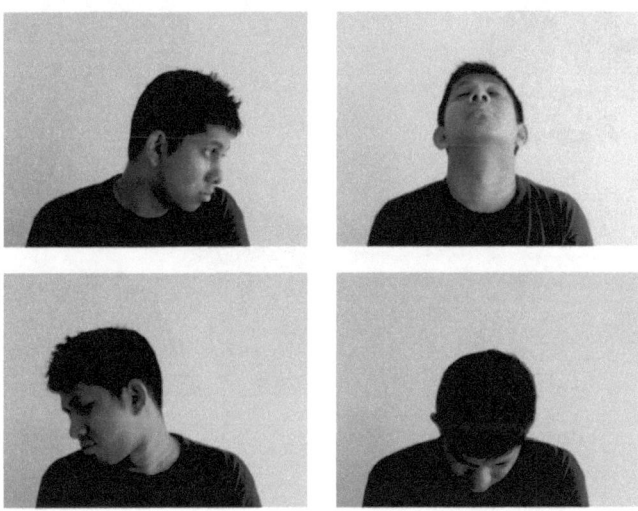

Figure 97 a,b,c,d

Slowly come out of this position and keep your head facing the center. Open your eyes wide and rotate your eyeballs ten times clockwise and ten times counterclockwise.

Now, close your eyes, and rub your palms together to warm your hands. Cup them over your eyes, and feel the energy in your eyes.

Open your eyes and join your hands together in the middle of your chest. As you inhale, push your palms and fingers together. As you exhale, join the tips of your fingers together, moving the palms away from each other. Repeat this ten times, remembering to inhale and exhale.

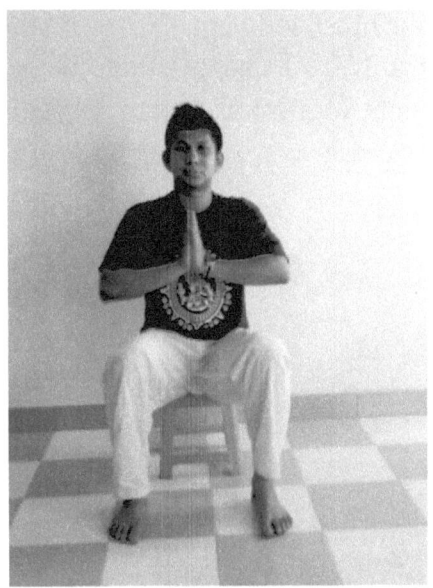
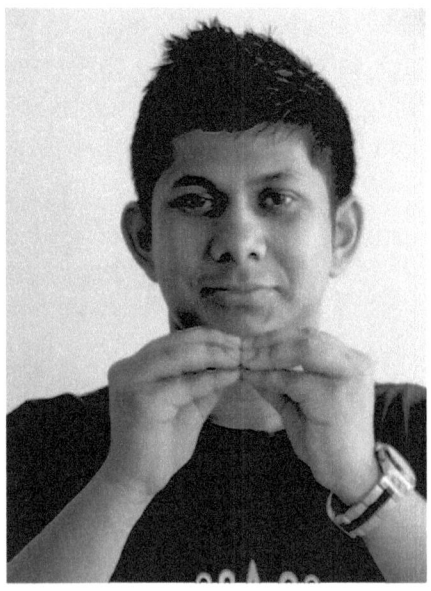

Figure 98   Figure 99

Slowly drop your hands to your thighs, make a fist with your right hand, and use your left hand to grab your right forearm. Rotate the right wrist ten times clockwise and ten times counterclockwise. Afterward, switch arms and do the same with your left wrist.

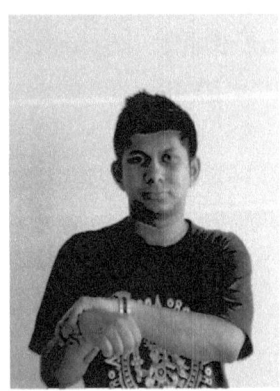
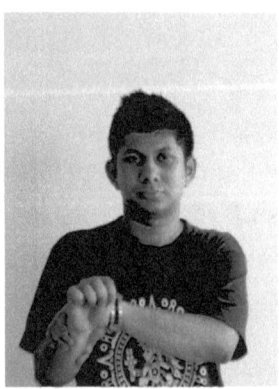
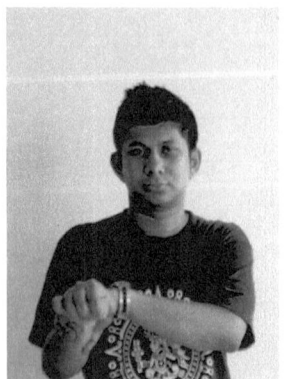

Figure 100 a,b,c

Now we will rotate our fingers. One at a time, rotate each finger ten times clockwise and ten times counterclockwise. Start with your right thumb and continue until you've rotated all fingers on each hand.

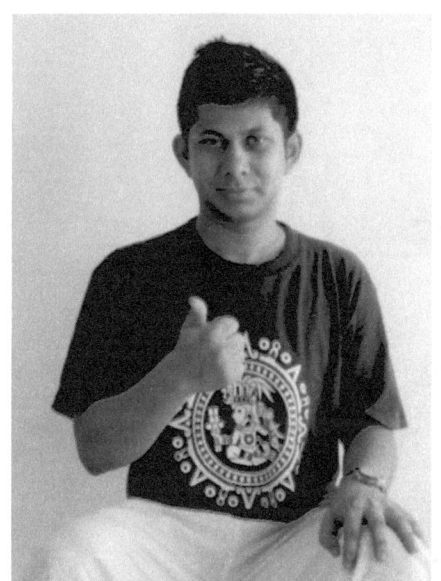 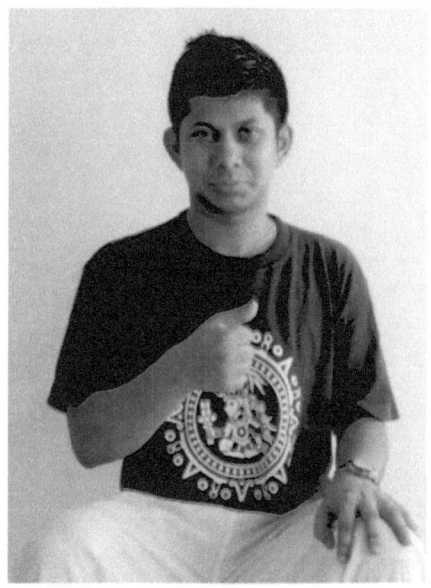

Figure 101 a,b

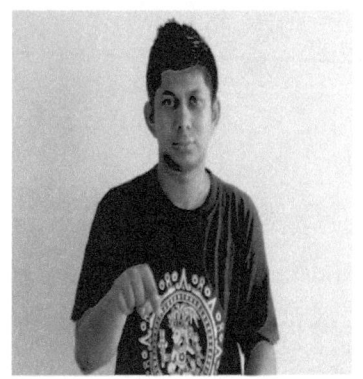 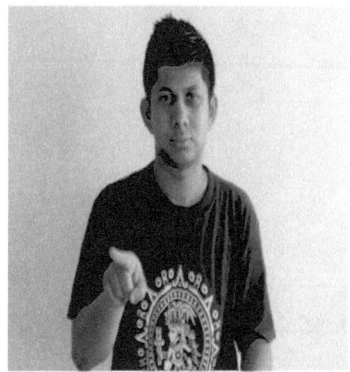

Figure 102 a,b

A better Life with Parkison's

Improving your Facial Expression, Swallowing, and Drooling (Face Yoga)

Push your lips out as though you are kissing the air, like a pig's face.

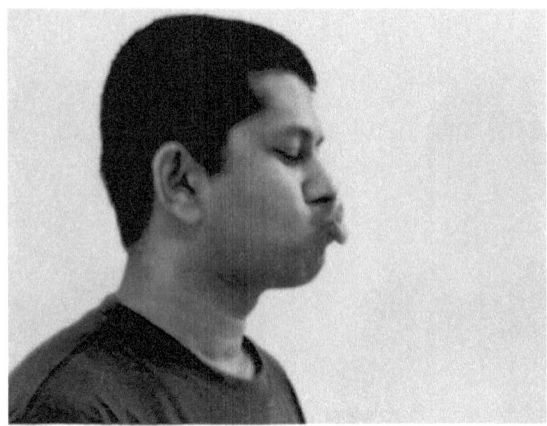

Figure 103

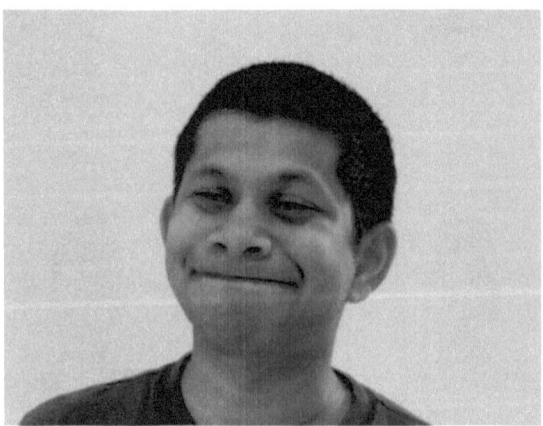

Figure 104

Now make the face like a chimpanzee by turning down your lower lip.

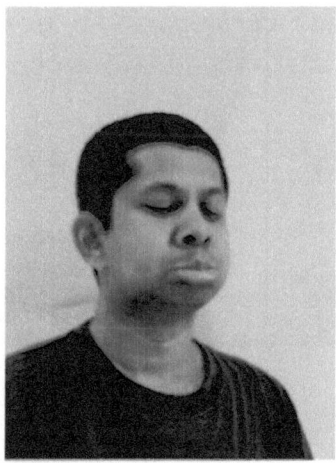

Figure 105

Next, make a face like a rabbit by pushing your upper teeth out, and act as though you're eating a carrot.

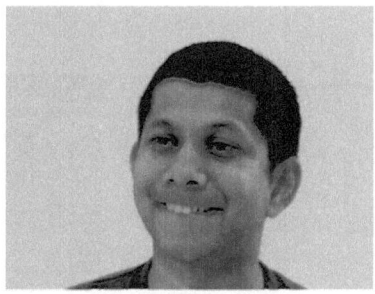

Figure 106

Let your tongue loll out of your mouth like a dog, breathing deeply.

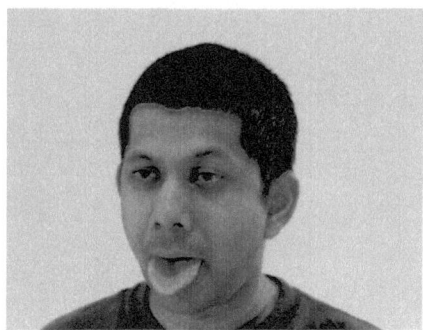

Figure 107

Make strange faces, and allow yourself to play with your eyes, lips, cheeks, nose, tongue, and ears. Allow your body to make noises

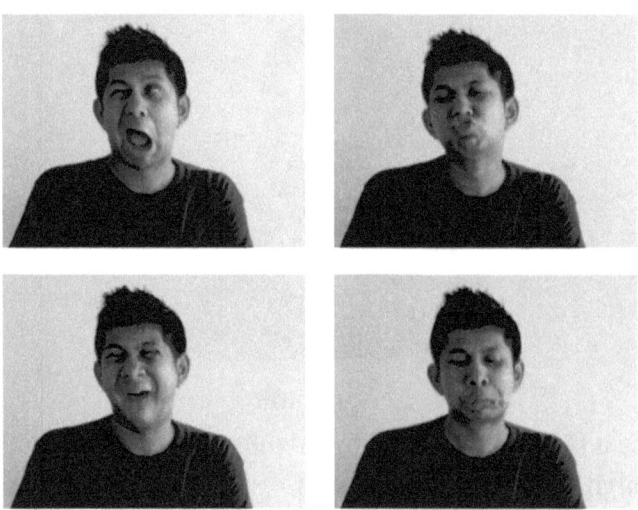

Figure 108 a,b,c,d

as you rotate your tongue inside your mouth and

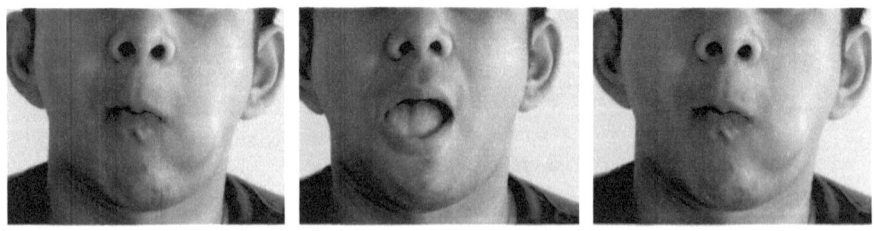

Figure 109 a,b,c

then do the same with your tongue outside your mouth.

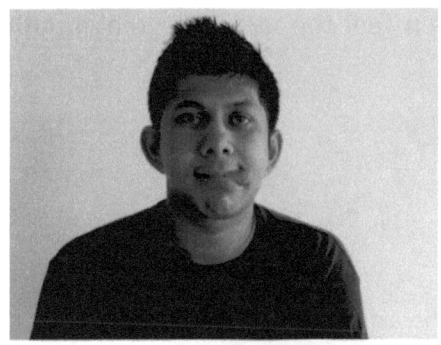 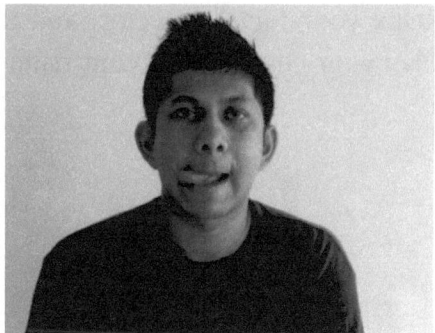

Figure 110 a,b

Vibrate your lips, creating a motorcycle-like sound.

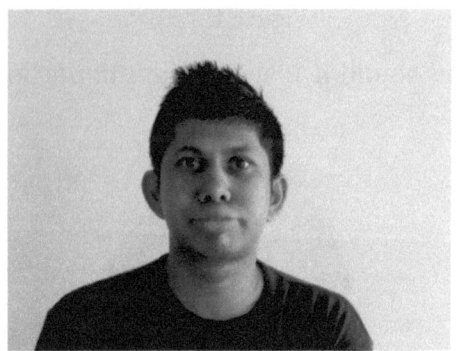

Figure 111

Improve by adding finger and play with your lips like a child.

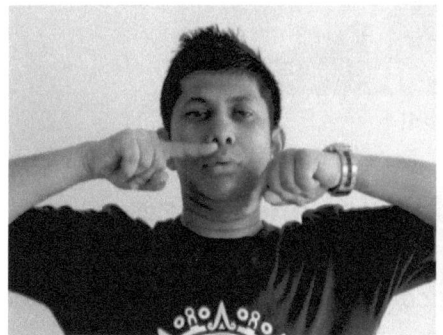 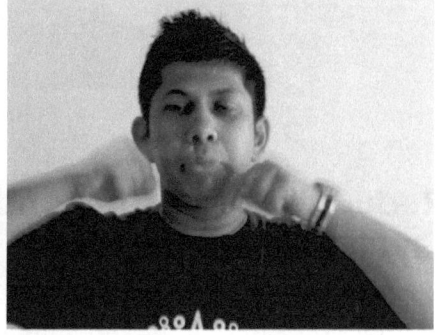

Figure 112 a,b

Relax your facial muscles, and then feel the air with your mouth. Clap your cheeks with your palms.

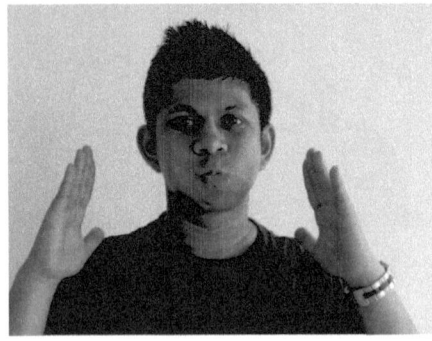 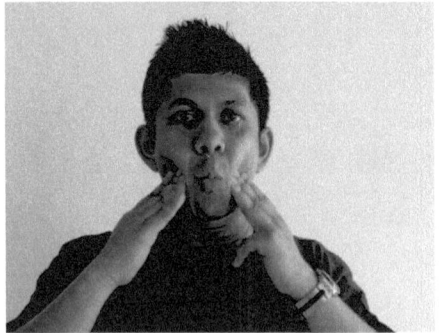

Figure 113 a,b

Next, whistle. The sound it makes is less important than the facial movements.

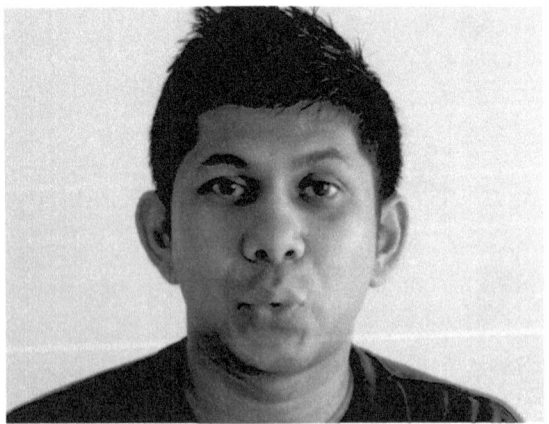

Figure 114

Reducing Depression and Improving Voice Quality (Laughter Yoga)

Laugh with your abdomen, and place your hand over your abdomen so that you can feel the movement as you do so. *Ha ha ha.*

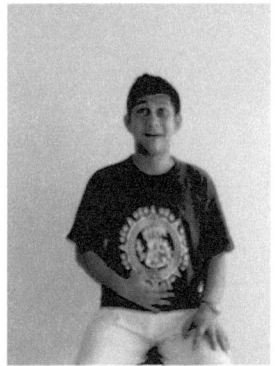

Figure 115

Laugh with your chest, and feel the movement of your lungs. *Ha ha ha.*

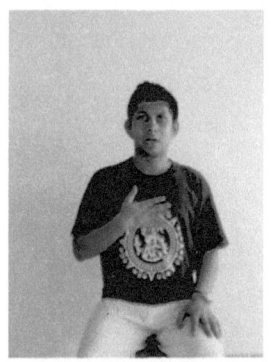

Figure 116

Now laugh with your throat. *Ho ho ho.*

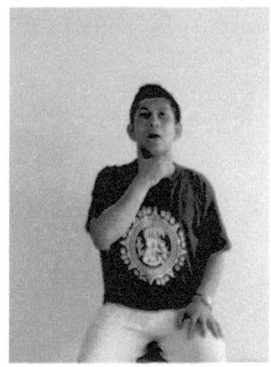

Figure 117

Laugh with your mouth.

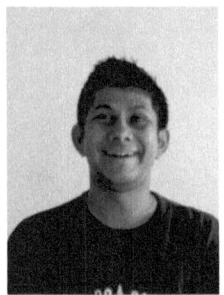

Figure 118

Then laugh with your nose. Open your eyes, and laugh spontaneously, naturally. *Ha ha ho ho hee hee hee.* Spread your legs and hands, and allow laughter to consume your entire body.

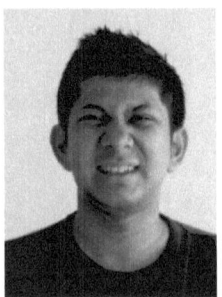

Figure 119

Open your eyes, and laugh spontaneously, naturally. *Ha ha ho ho hee hee hee.* Spread your legs and hands, and allow laughter to consume your entire body.

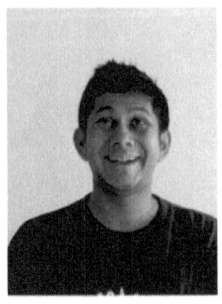

Stress Management (Yoga Breathing)

Sit in a comfortable posture in your chair. Straighten your spine, head, and neck.

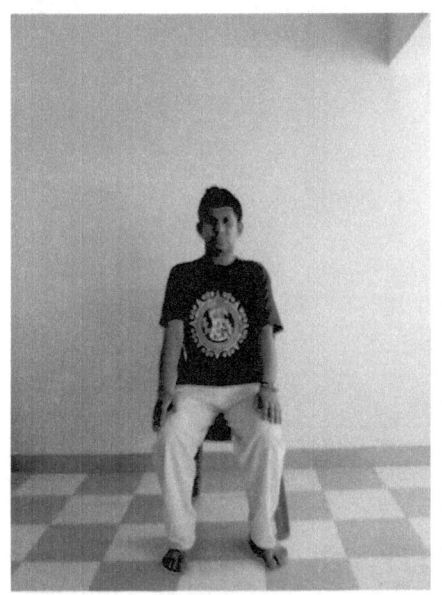

Figure 120

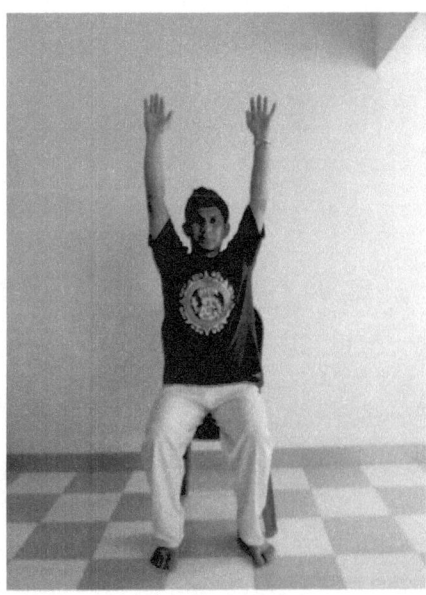

Figure 121

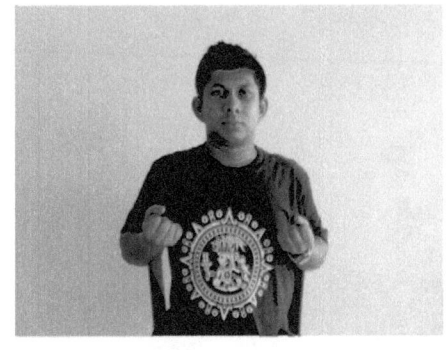

Figure 122

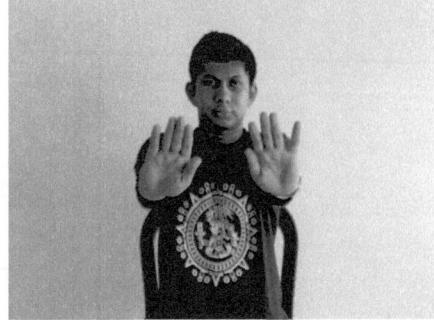

Figure 123

Using your index fingers, close one nostril at a time to practice alternate nostril breathing. First close the right nostril with the right hand's index finger, and inhale through the left nostril. Then close the left nostril as you open the right, and exhale through your right nostril. Alternate so that you inhale through your right nostril and exhale through the left. Repeat this ten times, ensuring that your lips are closed and that your inhalations are deep and long.

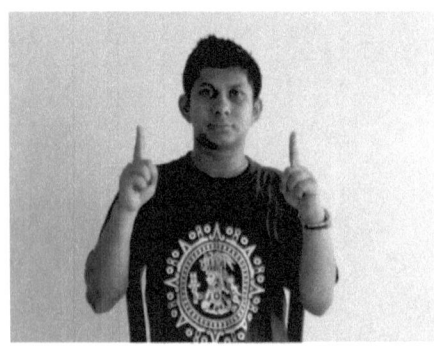

Figure 124

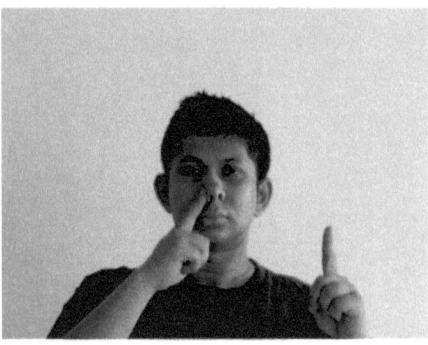

Figure 125

Inhale through your nose and then plug your ears with your index fingers. As you exhale, keep your lips closed and hum like a humming bee. Repeat this breathing pattern ten times before slowly dropping your hands back to your sides.

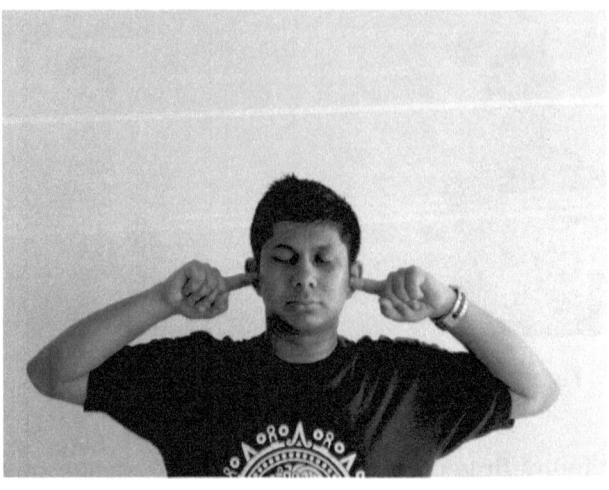

Figure 126

Improving Cognitive Function (Meditation)

Now we will do a meditation using finger coordination to relax your mind and feel the peace within. We will coordinate our fingers as we chant: A, U, M, E. Join the thumb and the index finger and say "A," then the middle finger and say "U," and the ring finger and say "M," and on the small finger, say "E." Keep your eyes closed and your hands on your thighs with your palms facing up. A-U-M-E. A-U-M-E. Repeat this ten times.

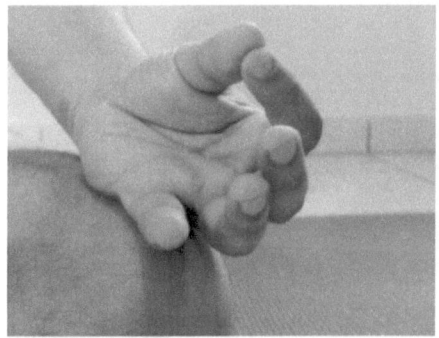
Figure 127

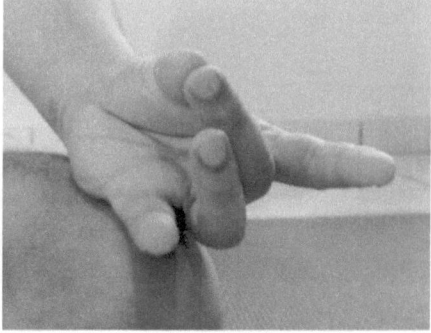
Figure 128

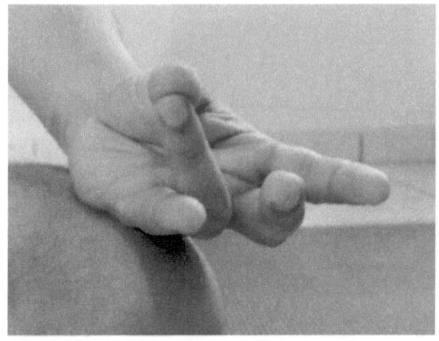
Figure 129

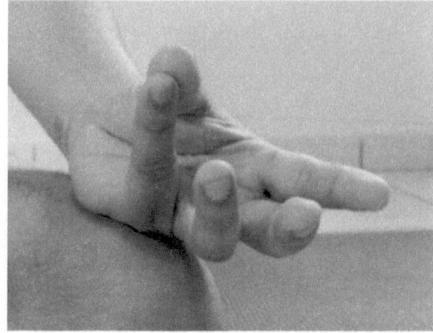
Figure 130

Keep your eyes closed and feel the peace within. Smile with your eyes, lips, and cheeks until your whole face is smiling. Smile with your whole body, and as you focus on your happiness, allow your mind and soul to smile as well.

Slowly open your eyes and come out of the meditation. This yoga session is complete.

One can mix both Yoga I and Yoga II exercises based on need and interest.

This Parkinson's yoga can be more individualized based on the specific needs of the practitioner. One can contact the author for more information about modifications.

PART 3 –
SELF HELP

Self help is the best help. No one can help a person who does not take an active role in his or her own wellbeing.

Chapter 8: Practical Solutions for Parkinson's Patients

Coping with tremors:

Remember that no control is the best control. Do not try to control the tremor. Accept the tremor, and feel it with love. It's like a special dance. There are many ways to reach your goal. If you want to lift a cup but have a tremor in your right hand, use the left. If necessary, use your mouth to bring the cup nearer to you.

If you're sitting in a public place, don't feel ashamed that your needs are different than others. Don't feel the need to hide your tremors.

You can also hold the part of your body that has the tremor, or use humming bee breathing and deep abdominal breathing to relax the brain.

Managing stiffness:

Whenever you stretch your muscles, push, twist or turn your body, you must exhale. Practice implementing the movements in this book without stressing your muscles. Don't think of movements as right or wrong; simply imagine the movements if necessary. Any movements you make towards yoga therapy are a success.

Yoga dancing and Parkinson's:

Yoga has a deep connection with dancing, as dancing means the expression of your inner feelings and rhythm with movements. *Yoga* means "to connect." When your expressions, rhythm, and movement are connected to your body, mind, emotions, and soul at the same time, that is yoga dancing. Dance freely to music without thinking about getting the steps right or what others may think.

If you are sitting in a wheel chair and cannot walk, you can still dance with your shoulders, hands, and facial expressions. If you're bedridden, meditate on dancing; there is still power in imagining these movements.

Ways to get up and turn to the side:

Sometimes, patients find it difficult to stand after sitting or lying down, and sometimes it can be difficult to shift over to your side. Think of your body like a rocking chair. If you're sitting on a chair, sit towards the front, and then rock your body forward and backwards, using this momentum to throw your body up without putting weight onto your knees. Instead of relying on your knees, support yourself with your lower back. The same can be done when lying in bed.

In order to turn on your side in bed, bend your legs and bring both the knees to the chest. Keep your hands on your knees while exhaling, and turn to the side. If you cannot turn on your own, imagine doing so in your mind. It will motivate you in the long run and help you get to the point where you can turn on your own without needing help.

Help with walking:

Inhale on one step and exhale on the next, practicing breathing exercises and coordinating your breath with your walking.

Go for a walk in morning and evening in a park that is free from dust and smoke. Others who are unable to go out may want to practice in an open place or in a room with fresh air. The body must be straight while walking. Keep your head, neck, and spine aligned. Inhale slowly and deeply, maintain a rhythm as you step. Count to four steps as you inhale, and count to six as you exhale.

If necessary, you may need to start by inhaling over the course of two steps and exhaling over the next two steps. With some practice, you can reach four steps for inhaling and six for exhaling.

Once you've mastered this, try counting to eight steps as you inhale and twelve steps as you exhale. Finally, once you're comfortable enough to do so, count to twelve steps as you inhale and eighteen as you exhale. If you're able to do this, you may not need to count your steps any longer. Simply practice taking rhythmic steps and breathing in this pattern. After two to three years of practice, you may be able to do this for about an hour without pause.

This method of walking while thinking about your breath will improve your ability to walk and help you avoid freezing. Do not think about freezing or hold your breath; instead, just walk and count as you inhale and exhale.

Improving swallowing:
Do face yoga (see the sections for face yoga in Yoga I and Yoga II)

Falling:
Fall like a baby or like a cat; loosen your limbs rather than freezing and stiffening your limbs. If possible, catch onto something or find another way to break your fall, but do not stress. Relax your muscles.

Martial arts practices like Jijitsu and Akido teach more about how to fall, and these are worth studying if you're interested in knowing more about how best to fall without hurting yourself. Just remember that after every fall, we stand back up more straight. Failure teaches more things than success.

Depression:
Do laugh yoga and face yoga when you are depressed (See Yoga I or Yoga II)

Pain and mental agony:

If you concentrate on your pain, it will only get worse. Mother Earth suffers from the pains of storms, oil drilling, and natural calamities, but Mother Earth is not disturbed.

Instead of thinking about the part of your body that is in pain, focus on other sensations. Think about how other parts of your body are feeling. What sounds can you hear? What is your breathing like? What does the touch of your clothes feel like? Engage with the thousands of other things happening at the same moment, and concentrate on the flow of these other feelings.

This can be difficult to master, but it can be made easier by listening to music or talking to others about their problems. This will give you something to focus on besides your own pain and allow you to engage with others. You can also cultivate a new hobby, like painting or joining a star-watching group. Having other things on which you can focus your mind will help you gain more control over how your attention is divided.

Problem Management

Parkinson's is a movement disorder, so every day, patients should practice Yoga I (Yoga for mobile patients) or Yoga II (Yoga for immobile patients) for better quality of movement. This will improve quality of life in turn. Some of the problems patients face everyday can be managed like this:

a) **Small Steps** - When we learn walking in our childhood, we do not think much about our walking – we just walk. So when it is difficult to walk, don't think about it as a Parkinson's symptom. Instead, just think about walking. Inhale, and take a step. Exhale, and take another step. Step on the lines between tiles or floorboards, if possible, to increase coordination and give you something on which to focus.

b) **Freezing** – When a Parkinson's patient freezes, his or her metabolism changes rapidly. If we can slow down or balance this metabolism, then we can manage freezing. Do not try to force movement when freezing. Just take a long deep inhalation, exhale very slowly, and hold the breath as long as is comfortable. Then inhale again, and repeat this sequence five more times. Slowly, try to return to natural movements.

   Another technique is to kneel and walk on your knees before trying to stand. You can also take a few sideways steps and then restart your normal walking patterns.

c) **Tremors** - Suppose that your right hand shivers, making it difficult to write. When the tremors start, don't try to control it with your brain; just accept that it's happening. Hold the tremoring part of your body with a non-tremoring hand, and focus on abdominal breathing (Yoga I).

d) **Drooling & swallowing problems** – Whenever saliva comes out of your mouth, whistle as many times as you can. Don't worry about whether you're making any sound; just blow the air out for better swallowing capability. Follow this by performing face yoga, focusing particularly on tongue movements.

e) **Standing up from a chair** - One can use the Rock & Roll movement to stand up. Rock in the chair a little, and use the momentum of rocking to propel your body into a standing position.

f) **Depression** – Do laugh yoga for at least half an hour. Aim to laugh for half an hour every day. Make a laughing club with your family and friends to meet together on the weekends and laugh.

Chapter 9: Clinical Procedure

Once, I asked my professor, "Why did you bring Ayurvedic therapy and yoga into a German hospital?" Though Ayurveda is accepted as wellness method in Europe and American hotels, there are so many other forms of medicine available, so why use these?

He answered, "After practicing neurology for forty years, I saw the limitations of modern medicine. Modern medicine is good for surgery and antibiotics, but for a total lifestyle disease like Parkinson's, treatment with drugs alone can't give you the best results. That's why I became interested in complimentary medicine, specifically Ayurveda and yoga."

Yoga and Ayurveda have demonstrated their healing power time and again, but this cannot always be objectively studied, as many forms of medicine would like to be.

Presently there are no medical gadgets to measure many of the effects of Yoga and Ayurveda. Still, some improvements can be measured.

When patients first came to us at the hospital, we would do a colonoscopy to evaluate the condition of their large bowels. After they ate Ayurvedic food, primarily following a Ayurvedic-vegan diet for twenty-one days, the large intestine was again examined.

Measurements could also be taken with the smell test. When patients first arrived for treatment, they would undergo a smell test. After Ayurvedic treatment to the nose in order to improve brain function, they would repeat the test. We were able to measure that their ability to identify smells increased after Ayurvedic treatment.

Concept of therapy & infrastructure of the Neurology & Complemnatry clinic

Now that people are coming to recognize the limitations of modern medicine, it's becoming more apparent that conventional methods are not adequately effective for treating chronic diseases. As a result, interest has shifted towards complementary medical methods. Complementary medicine means that two medical systems are used simultaneously, such as Modern medicine and Ayurveda & Yoga. The Ayurvedic & Yoga method, which has been around for over five thousand years, was used alongside conventional medicine for our patients. In the clinic, modern technical gadgets were used in the diagnosis and treatment process. Then Ayurvedic and yoga therapies were used for treatment along with modern medicine.

Yoga and Ayurvedic medicine operate on the principle that Parkinson's disease starts at an early stage in a region of the olfactory organ and the gastrointestinal tract. The gastrointestinal disturbances start at least twelve years preceding the motor disorders. This is also consistent with the views of modern medical treatments, which have used detoxifying measures and L-dopa-containing preparations as inner medicine for many years. By drawing on the Ayurvedic experience, the hospital successfully treats the olfactory disorders and disorders of the gastrointestinal tract. Since it is generally assumed that the majority of Parkinson's disease cases are caused by a genetic component and a chronic intoxication develops as a result, the clinic tried to tackle the toxic component, especially as the genetic cause is not thought to be currently treatable.

According to Ayurvedic medical thinking, the imbalance in the body's energies result in toxins, which contribute significantly to the emergence of chronic diseases. The clinic gave detoxification massages, steam therapy, therapeutic enemas and nasal detoxification based on the varying diagnoses and patient needs.

Our clinic staffed three neurologists, two general doctors, two Ayurvedic doctors, a dietician, ten experienced nurses, a yoga teacher, eight therapists, and a psychologist.

Our ward had forty beds and a common dining place. It was equipped with spaces for playing indoor games so that patients could improve fine motor skills as well. We held tango lessons so that patients could improve balance skills, and in the Yoga Hall, patients could enjoy massages and practice yoga with their peers.

Chapter 10: Letters From Patients

My patients sometimes gave me their photos or music CDs, and often they sent me letters and cards.

With their permission, I would like to share some of these notes with you in this book.

Whenever I read these letters, I feel grateful to be a part of their healing processes.

I would like to thank Mr. Ray for the excellent yoga exercises. I will continue to practice them at home.
—Hans

Raja Ray introduced me to yoga, which I will never forget. Western people need yoga.
In gratitude,
-Wolfgang

Mr. Raja Ray has helped me through yoga. Over a span of two and a half weeks, I've gotten better (my steps are getting bigger) and my balance has also improved significantly. My speech and articulation are again clear. My facial expressions have improved significantly, and my breathing is much better.
Mr. Ray was able to pass his knowledge along very well. I am obliged to him.
With greatest thanks,
-Eckart

Mr. Ray has massaged me to the finest. Now, I'm re-mobilized. His style of yoga has also benefited me. I am eager to answer any further questions on the book that he is writing. I wish him success in his future life cycle.
-Gernot

I was desperate and went very crooked,
that was the Raja Ray with his charm,
He took out his oil pot and made the oil warm,
Massaged me from head to foot and arm.
Day after day must go the way
now I can stand up straight again.
Also the yoga, what he taught me,
is worth praise.
I wish you all the best in all your account
and good health.
- In gratitude---
Friedhlem

I am sure that yoga will help me better to move my joints, increase my overall agility, and achieve a peaceful balance. Thanks to Ray Raja, who made me familiar with yoga. I'll stick with it.
-Karl Dieter

Yoga and an Ayurvedic diet will be an integral part of my life.
Mr. Ray has shown me the way. I thank you.
-Arthur

Dear Radja,
I like to look at my health breaks in the Protestant hospital in Hattingen. Encounters with people will particularly stick in my memory.

Your personal care, which was marked by patience and serenity, greatly impressed me. I will always remember the way you took me under your yoga wing.

I already look forward to my next stay in Hattingen and a reunion with you. To you personally, of course I wish all the best. Until then, your patient, who forgets again and again to close his eyes.
- Manfred

Dear Raja,
During my stay in Hattingen's Protestant Hospital at Neurology 1 and Complementary Medicine Department, Prof. H. Przuntek significantly improved the human atmosphere. The treatments with the Ayurvedic diet and facility requirements for my well-being were wonderful

Through exercises for physical and mental fitness, I met you, dear Raja. Your style of yoga exercises with multiple participants and the detoxification massage like Abhyanga were of great help. The way you guided and explained yoga to me was a delight!

But I do not want to leave out one particular event. On Tuesday, shortly before the end of my treatment, I told you that I had felt a pulled muscle in my right shoulder and arm for years. You pulled my arm very firm and quickly, just like that, and you said "The soreness is now gone!"
The soreness really disappeared!
-Rolf

Dear Raja Ray!
You are so present in yoga that I succeed again and again at being in the here and now, and in my body. Wonderful!
Your inner light has taken me.
Heartfelt thanks! – Barbara

Dear Raja,
It would be wonderful if there were records of your singing the Hymns. Make a CD, perhaps even an entire session!

Perhaps you can advise me as to whether it's possible to attend your yoga sessions as an outpatient.

- Kristina

Dear Raja Ray,
You, with your quiet way, have helped me turn my head off! Yoga has helped me very much, and I will continue to do it at home.

Now I feel much more energy. Much obliged! I really hope that I can be here again next year.

- Margit

Dear Raja Ray,
When I entered the hospital, I was full of doubts, and I wondered if there was any sense to these strange concepts of Ayurveda and yoga.

Today, on the last day, I must say that I've come back like a newborn again in my return to everyday life. And you have played an essential role in that!!!

Thank you for that!

-Werner

Conclusion

It is difficult to communicate about Parkinson's management through a book. Parkinson's is a total body disease, and it takes many years to develop. Direct interaction is required to get connected and communicate all that I've learned and learning about it.

Yoga and Ayurveda gives one a different outlook on life, and it helps you find new body movements and thought processes.

In the future, I will try to make workshops about Parkinson's yoga to interact directly with more Parkinson's patients. I also want to share more information about how to cook healthy, tasty food that taps into the inner potential and healing of our bodies, with Ayurveda principles and concepts.

It took many years to write this book after working full-time in the hospital and learning German in a foreign country. It was difficult to find time to sit and write, but my patients and friends gave me the motivation to do so. I still teach and learn from my Parkinson's patients.

Please feel free to ask or recommend about Parkinson therapies, Ayurveda, Yoga and further improvements about this book.

Whatever I am developing and learning, I hope to share it with you all in the future.

Regards & Namaste.
Raja Ray
Email- hatyog@gmail.com

About the Author

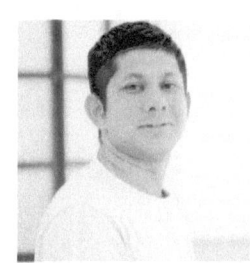

Raja Ray was born in Serampore, India. He learned to swim in the river Ganges, climbed & played in coconut tree ; trekked &climbed in Himalayan mountains from early childhood with his family. As his father hobby was mountaineering and also a banker by profession.

He learned about yoga, Ayurveda and Indian philosophy from his mother. She was a math teacher and also his headstand teacher. Raja graduated with a degree in literature, history and philosophy from Calcutta University.

From his early childhood days he visited many ashrams, getting to know many yogis, sadhus and swamis. After studying and finishing his teacher training and Ayurveda Panchakarma in Kerala, he lived in Ashram. There were offers to become a monk, but he loved traveling and worked at the bank for a while. But that was not his area. He worked with many Medical doctors and healers from different traditions, In Kolkata,Kerala and Goa.

He has practiced yoga for 26 years and teaches yoga, Ayurveda and Meditation for the last 12 years.

Presently he is working with a Leading Ayurveda Institute in Germany.

Literature

1. *Yoga-Therapie.* Gesund und leistungsfähig durch Yoga und Ayurveda - A.G Mohan

2. *Asana, Pranayama, Mudra and Bandha:* Swami Satyananda Saraswati

3. *Yoga as Therapeutic Exercise:* A Practical Guide for Manual Therapist - Luise Woerle

4. *Yogic Management Of Common Diseases:* Swami Karmananda

5. *Yoga and Medical Science:* Dr Krishna Raman

6. *Parkinson's Disease:* A Complete Guide for Patients and Families by William J. Weiner MD (Author), Lisa M. Shulman MD (Author), Anthony E. Lang MD FRCP (Author)

7. *Horst Przuntek / Thomas Müller (eds.):* Diagnosis and Treatment of Parkinson's Disease - State of the Art

8. *Wolfgang H. Oertel/Günther Deuschl/Werner Poewe:* Parkinson-Syndrome und andere Bewegungsstörungen

9. *P. Riederer / D.B. Calne / R. Horowski / Y. Muzuno / C.W. Olanow / E. Poewe / M.B.H. Youdim (eds.):* Advances in Research on Neurodegeneration

10. *Claudia Trenkwalder:* Parkinson - Die Krankheit verstehen und bewältigen

www.ingramcontent.com/pod-product-compliance
Lightning Source LLC
Chambersburg PA
CBHW020425220526
45464CB00002B/572